Tricky Cervix

Written by Mary Manning

This book is not medical advice. This is a true story of one woman trying to conceive, a crappy path of infertility and menopause, and her quest to normalize it all.

CHAPTER ONE

ACT I

When you purchase ovulation kits and pregnancy tests in bulk, there is a problem. The normal, healthy, couple takes up to one year to conceive; that is twelve attempts. Twelve. That sounds so easy. Hindsight.

It is Halloween, 2010. Children dress up and parents take pictures. I wonder what will be our child's first costume. Most likely a vegetable, peas are popular, or maybe baby Yoda, or baby-old person.

Facebook and social media are packed with pictures of friends' children dressed up and looking adorable. No one ever publically posts that they are infertile and crushed when they see a child. April fool's day though, may be the worst social media holiday for the infertile; (besides Mother's Day) why would anyone think being pregnant is a joke? My feed was inundated with photos of positive pregnancy tests or sonogram images taunting me, only to be a: *we got you!* Hilarious.

I am sick of waiting. I am sick of trying to conceive. How much longer do we have to try? Why does my body suck? Why is Tim, my husband, so calm? When will he quit smoking? Why can un-wanting, unhealthy, jobless, UFO sighting, paper-bag Boone's Farm ZIMA drinking people get pregnant?!

When will I be kind, and non-judgmental?

Rewind

In July of 2006 Tim and I begin talking about a family. We had
always agreed we wanted kids, but now, we were ready to stop
trying *to not* try to have kids. We gave up the condoms and I
stopped my last pack of birth control pills.

It was a monumental experience. We were on the same page;
welcoming the idea of a child into our lives. We knew that we
would never be financially ready, so why give ourselves that
deadline? The goal was to work on our debt, buy a home, move
up in our careers and have a family. It was a simple checklist. I
had siblings with children, but Tim is the eldest in his family. We
were the first married of our immediate friends, so no one else
was even considering kids at this time, like us.

My gynecologist had given me a plan to *count days*. I would
count from the first day of my last period, fourteen days, then
within that time frame and when my cervical mucus lining was
like egg whites and stretchy, that was magic time. (This
insinuates that one should physically check said egg-white
stretchiness. Let's pause a moment; this instruction was given to
me as if it was routine that one examines her cervical mucus. This
was a surprise to me; I did not realize this was part of the female
hygienic regimen.) She also suggested not having intercourse
every day during the egg white time, but every other day. I
counted, I checked and we romped. I got my period and
attributed it to just having gotten off of the pill and my body
probably needed some time to re-adjust. I was certain it would
happen in no time, three of my four sisters had children and my
fourth sister was now trying.

In the months to follow Tim would have an accident at work that
would temporarily confine him to a wheelchair. I became his
caretaker for those months and needless to say, doing the deed
was not on my radar.

Once he was on the mend, we started trying again. I counted days, examined cervical mucus. Apparently stretching your cervical mucus between your fingers is not solely per a routine, but the initial method of determining ovulation. I saw another doctor and she gave me a temperature chart. I then start to take my basal body temperature every morning, in bed—before my feet even touch the floor as directed. I mark it on a paper chart, we have sex accordingly. After several unsuccessful months I move the data onto an Excel spreadsheet, as if our method of data mining will promote fertility. Next we begin with ovulation kits, readily available in grocery stores. One kit in particular was like a kids' chemistry set; you dip a litmus paper type strip into your pee and examine the color on the strip and compare it to the color on the bottle to determine when you have sex. It was a very involved method, and since we enjoyed traveling, it was not the most conducive to a discreet conception.

We keep trying, and my sister who had started trying when we did, had her first baby. At his baptism I couldn't stay for the whole ceremony. I was overcome with jealousy that I still had not gotten pregnant, and she did. Some of my family understood, but some did not. After all, no one really knew we were trying, and Tim had just suffered that terrible accident…

Jealousy is when you truly meet yourself. My salutation was tears. I wanted a baby. A simple thing…I mean, isn't that why I have had my period all these years; so one day I could have a baby?

Jealousy is described as suffering; you suffer when you lack something.

Are we doing it wrong?

Two years later, we purchase our first home, in 2008; we got to watch the Phillies win the World Series in our Craigslist furnished family room. It was our dream home and my mom (and pretty much everyone else) told me that once we settled into a home we would get pregnant in no time. This is when I learn that apparently all you need to do is *relax* and you will conceive. I decided to make another appointment and talk to my doctor about why I was still not pregnant. Everything about me on paper looked normal, they did a FSH test, and that too, was considered normal. This FSH test, follicle stimulating hormone test, is done on the third day of your period. It is a simple blood draw. But, this was a preliminary test; they were looking for numbers in what was a normal range. Spoiler alert, normal for one woman is not normal for another.

She said given that life was so hectic for me, to give it another year and see what happens. I spoke about how I seem to get so angry during my menstrual cycles and how crazy my skin breaks out with acne, but it seemed there was nothing safe to be done about either when trying to get pregnant. After all, to calm skin down and ease period discomfort one usually goes on birth control pills…yeah… I didn't press the issue with her, but accepted her diagnosis and went about doing the same crap we had been doing. What is the definition of insanity again?

I purchase ovulation kits in bulk and plead with Tim to do it every day. I make sex into a chore. It is a task on my check list and though I become open to trying new things, it really is only so I can get pregnant. I take every fun, every passion, every ounce of pleasure out of it and my sole purpose is to get that double line on a urine saturated stick. Feet in the air, ass on a pillow holding my body completely still, willing his sperm to seek, find, and burrow into my egg. I am sexy. I research what foods promote fertility, we eat them-- what positions promote conception, we do them… Sex becomes not sexy.

After what feels like my millionth period, I get another *not pregnant*. What the hell? Even, scratch off tickets say, *sorry, try again*.

I started going to the gynecologist in college, once the whole sex thing started. According to my mom, you don't have sex until you are married. So, being a good Catholic girl, I had sex with my college boyfriend and simply did not tell her. I used the college health center to get an appointment.

I remember being examined by my gynecologist, and she never alluded to me being different. I think every woman's fear is that our privates are wrong. Look wrong, are set up wrong or have some bizarre condition that we simply are not aware of. Frankly, I have never seen my own vagina nor seen any other woman's. Well…there was that girl in Arts High School who showed me her clitoris ring, but I was so shocked that she accessed herself so quickly in the girls bathroom near the sink that I did not really look at what she looked like, so I had no reference if mine looked different. And what partner in their right mind while in the act of intimacy is going to tell you that your vagina is a bit different from the other women?

So I went about my life thinking my vulva, vagina and all other inside parts were perfect. My experienced husband would eventually tell me if my parts were wrong. Right?

Do gynecologists compare aesthetic notes on patient vaginas? Am I on the hairy, smelly list?

In March of 2010 I get on Tim's case that he should have his sperm tested. We are now at four years of unprotected sex. He came home with his analysis. Low motility. I cried. Later that night our friends gave birth to their first son. We had approached the time of friends getting married and starting their families; they had caught up with us, and now we were married 5 years, we were behind.

Low motility sounds kind of cute, though…aw, your swimmers need swimmies…

In May of 2010 I had another gynecology appointment with a different doctor. I had to change insurances during the time previous, so I was making the rounds for my annual appointments. I told the doctor that I had been trying to start a family and wanted to know if I should begin the testing that would tell us more about what was wrong. I told him about Tim's test but that I wanted to know if there was anything else. He told me *clean living* was the key and gave me a referral to a fertility clinic.

Clean living was no alcohol, no drugs, healthy diet, exercise and managing stress appropriately. (Remember all those fat, high school girls smoking and drinking under the bridge? How the hell did they get pregnant?)   I made the appointment as soon as possible which was the end of July 2010. The night before the appointment Tim and I argued. He felt that making the appointment for us was a sign of giving up, that I had grown impatient and was ready to try the first procedure they recommended. I was so angry, but admitted to him, that my real reason for making the appointment was that I wanted the fertility doctors to scare him straight. He was the problem, he needed to quit smoking, we both needed to stop drinking alcohol and Tim had to lose weight. He understood and together we went to the fertility clinic fully expecting that we did not meet the criteria of an infertile couple.

Prior to our first fertility clinic appointment we had paperwork. There was female paperwork and male paperwork. We entered that we had been having unprotected sex for four years, but actively trying for two—it was hard to say. We filled it out honestly. Apparently, four years of unprotected sex without a pregnancy is a long time.

We met with the doctor first. He asked us the same questions as on the paperwork, but as if he did not have the answers in front of him. Which I found frustrating, it prolonged the process—I wanted an answer in that office, I wanted a fix in that office. With all the information, he determined we would begin testing. He predicted we had *unexplained infertility* and that IUI or intrauterine insemination would be our route. I cried, right then and there. When my suffering dam is at capacity, only public crying releases it. I knew that we knew nothing, and now we were going to find out. We then were assigned to a case nurse and she made us a list of what we were to do next and a folder containing information on IUI; it was our homework. I had no idea our sex life would now require research, studying and documentation let alone all the testing; I would become a fertility student. I would later come to know that *unexplained infertility* was fancy doctor speak for: *We do not fucking know.*

The third day of my upcoming period I would do a FSH test again, a blood draw, followed by a transvaginal (ooo la la) ultrasound. Then on the fifth day of that same period a HSG or dye test. In the meantime both Tim and I would have routine blood work done. I was given a prescription for an antibiotic to take the night before the dye test. The HSG or hysterosalpingogram is a test to determine if there are any blockages within my tubes; a dye would be squirted up there while I was x-rayed and ta-da we would have an answer. It is as weird and simple as it sounds.

We left the office overwhelmed. Tim suggested that since we were going to be arriving at work late anyway, that we go to a diner and get some breakfast. It was perfect and I refrained from public crying. It was like a date for us. That diner would forever be referred to as the *Baby Doctor Diner*.

We went to work. Later that night at home I went on the clinic's website and read about all the procedures. My heart ached and my vagina winced, I think it cried too. I read about IUI, then, I read about IVF and think, ugh, I do not want to have to do that one, it sounds awful. I looked into our insurance, both online and in the handbook we had been given after open enrollment and it seemed that most infertility treatments, up to three attempts, were covered under our plan. This was a huge sigh of relief and gratitude. But, still, we did not know anything yet.

The financial burden of seeking fertility treatments is overwhelming. However, there are many grants and foundations

that can assist those who qualify. I have no first-hand knowledge
of how to apply for these grants or become a recipient of any
financial help towards treatments. What I do know is that the
clinic we went to had plenty of information to share on their
website, and even had a staff member assigned to that
department. The great fortune of our insurance coverage never
escaped me.

Vulnerable.

August 9th, 2010

To my baby,

There was a time I did not want you. A time of fear and shock. Simply afraid of what others would think and how in the world we would succeed. It was a dark time and I did not see clearly.

Now an ache. You are quite simply, an ache. A longing. Every month we try to make you. So far, every month we fail and I cry. I have learned I am the jealous type. I see you and me in every woman's life. I see you in wombs and strollers. On the street and in the news—I do not know you, but it is like you could be mine, and I ache. You are in my family, on Facebook statuses, in books, magazines and everywhere I turn.

I want the morning sickness, the cramps, the cravings, the giggles, the hope, and the dreams for you, the fat, and the swollen feet. I will loan you my body for as long as needed. I will take care of this home for you until you leave. Then I will love you. All the time. You already are the smartest, funniest, prettiest, loving, caring, special, wonderful, amazing, talented, peaceful being in the world! You already can be anything you want.

You are loved by a flawed mother. I recognize my faults and may I never pass them to you. I want you so badly. I weep in your absence. I sob, longing for you.

The hope of you fills me with joy—and I am doing all that I can so that you may join us. We have asked doctors for help and we are awaiting test results. I accept however you come into our lives. I accept who you are and who you become, no matter what. I accept your flaws and shortcomings. I accept that you will be a better person than I. I love you, though we have yet to meet.

Love,

Mom

On August 9th, 2010, I have my first FSH test and ultrasound with the fertility clinic. They check hormone levels in the blood and actually count follicles on an ultrasound. Follicles, meaning egg opportunities in your ovaries; you see your body forms follicles, but only shoots out one (sometimes two) egg(s) to await the sperm.

I had the test early in the morning and the rest of the day off from work. I drove to the clinic, scared, but got there safely. I wore a tampon, not realizing that a pad would have been the better choice. Rookie mistake.

I sat in the waiting room of the clinic expecting the best. I was a healthy young woman. I did not smoke, do drugs, I exercised regularly—was training for a marathon, and I was in a loving and monogamous relationship with my husband. I had had this blood test before, about a year before and my results had been normal, so I was expecting the same. My husband on the other hand, was a smoker and did little to no exercise and could stand to lose a few pounds. His tests showed low motility. I claimed it was because his sperm all had smokers lungs, and it is pretty hard to swim with a cough. With all of this knowledge I was confident while waiting alone in the mauve room. This test was simply a formality in my head, for Tim, clearly was the problem. Maybe these tests will scare him, he will quit smoking and we will get pregnant in no time!

I blamed Tim for our lack of children. I sat there awaiting tests, blaming my husband. Convinced it could not possibly have anything to do with me.

The nurse called me in and told me what I was to do. She had a shaved head and I felt an immediate kindred spirit to her—I had an Ani Difranco phase… I admitted that I was still wearing a tampon and she showed me where the bathroom was so that I could remove it. The bathroom at the clinic is homey; there is a shelf there with all your feminine needs. However, their choice of pad is strictly based on costs. This *is* your momma's pad. It is the old mattress type that on the commercials they dump blue dye on to show its absorbency. I have often thought that should they change the dye to red, but some may think that offensive. I find maxi pads that are comparable to diapers, offensive.

I head back into my exam room. I undress from the waist down and leave my socks on. I fold panties and jeans and place them on the chair near my purse, my sneakers on the floor. I hop on the table that has a giant rectangle pad on it with butcher paper underneath.   I place the disposable gyno exam napkin over my lap like a good patient and wait.

There is a knock, followed by my shaved head nurse and a doctor whom I have never met. He reminds me of a turtle, or if Jim Henson had an angry turtle gynecologist character who was so tired of looking at vaginas and just dreamed of being in show business.

I am instructed to put my feet in the stirrups and lie back. The lights are turned off and a cold condom-ed object is inserted. It is more awkward than uncomfortable. I wish that the three of us knew each other better—like we could joke about something to make the time spent together more pleasant.

I look at the monitor and see black. To me, there is nothing there, barren, empty with some sparse grey digitized movement. I am a bit relieved that there is not a lost and now found tampon from years back still up there.

"Well, here is your problem!" I imagine my turtle doctor saying.

"How old are you?" he asks. I am snapped back into reality.

"31." I reply, almost forgetting my own age.

He slips the wand from my body and there is heaviness in the room. He is writing something down and tells me they will call me that afternoon. The nurse does not look at me.

I ask, "Well, did everything look normal?"

"Eh, not too many eggs. They will call you."

I am told to get dressed and to sit on one of the chairs in the hall then they will draw my blood.

I get dressed in my big huge diaper of a pad generously given to me, certainly worth the co-pay, and my pulse and thoughts race. What did he mean, not too many eggs? Am I out of eggs? Can they see that? I tear up, and stop myself from crying; I reassure myself, and like a mantra I repeat; they are gathering information, we will know more after today. It sinks in, and I am terrified that I could be the problem.

I sit in the hallway, silently begging that they take my blood already so I can hurry to the car and cry out dramatically, *not too many eggs!?* I see my shaved head nurse with other patients and I swear she is looking at me like I am the dirty, kennel cough puppy no one will adopt. Like she knows something grave, and will tell me all about it this afternoon.

My blood is quickly drawn and as promised I head to my car and cry. It is a ridiculous cry because it is based solely on my anxiety. I straighten myself out and head home. Tim is still there, he has not left for work yet. I walk in upset and tell him what happened. He begins to discount what happened, telling me that *some lab tech* told me that, and what does he know? I then explained that it was an actual doctor who gave the exam.

He hugged me and said, "Not too many eggs compared to what?"

I spend much of the day crying, wondering what it all means. I talk to my mom and she tells me to stay positive and that she is praying for me.

I decide to eat and watch trash TV to get my mind off the unknown, when the phone rings. It is my doctor, who is luckily not the turtle doctor. He tells me my test result and ultrasound was not encouraging. I need to do more blood tests. My prolactin level was very high, my FSH was elevated and my follicle count was quite low. I cried right there, on my kitchen steps, into the phone even though I had no idea what that all meant. Honestly, *not encouraging* was all I heard.

"Hang in there, kid." He said, and then he hung up.

A few minutes later my case nurse called, she talked me through the next steps. Explaining that I needed to do another blood test, this time fasting and no nipple stimulation.

What? Nipple stimulation?

She is very clear about the nipple stimulation part…I didn't recall any previous nipple stimulation prior to the blood test, but okay, no nipple stimulation. Got it.

I asked her about the egg count and she admitted that they saw only four follicles. A normal woman has ten to twelve. She kindly said what I was thinking; that she was sorry that this was happening and that it is frustrating to feel you take one step forward and three steps back. We hang up, and I would get Labcorp orders in the mail soon to retest my prolactin level with no nipple stimulation later that week. She also instructs me to not have the dye test this cycle, but repeat the prolactin test and then on my next period, on day three we will repeat the FSH test and do the dye test that month. I take a lot of notes during this phone call. So, essentially another month needs to go by. It felt like someone had moved the finish line right before I was about to get there.

I cried. The wailing, sobbing, Nancy Kerrigan *WHY ME* cry.

I called Tim and all I said was, "They called, and there is a problem, and it is me."

"I will be home soon; I will leave here as soon as I can."

There are no words to describe this type of crying. It is a sadness of unbelievable strength, yet, when it was out, I felt better. I could move on. Then, something would trigger another round of sobbing—for example, a commercial for auto insurance.

I called my mom, I wrote in my journal, I cried and Tim hugged me whenever I needed it. Our dog cuddled and licked my face, and I am pretty sure I had ice cream.

I Google prolactin. Now that, is hilarious…more on that later…

I get my blood drawn to repeat the prolactin test and once again, my levels are elevated along with an antithyroglobulin. Huh?

We wait some more. Since I am to repeat my FSH tests again on my next menstrual cycle I decide to change my mind set.

I realize that I have a physical manifestation of how stress kills. I have spent my years worried. Worrying about work, money, love, family and everything else in between. My body is literally saying—stop, you need a break, you are all messed up despite what you perceive! Slow down. Calm down!

I have the luxury of taking a week off from work; (because I can never take off during the semesters, I work most weekends with no compensation and I have built a bank of unused leave) I book a massage and plan to do only happy things. I tell almost everyone that I am like a rubber band ready to snap and need some time off. The truth is I am a rubber band that has been stretched too far and I am actually unable to snap, I am dry and withered—I will break and no one will know, my break will impact no one. I am the old, dry, cracked remnant of a rubber band in the junk drawer, milling about with ketchup, soy sauce packets and a bent paper clip.

I visit family, I share my story with my four sisters and I seek counseling among my friends. I let Tim love me, and I get a library card. I do things for myself, things that seem silly, but necessary.

Day one of my next period I call the fertility clinic to schedule my FSH tests and HSG. I make the appointments while at work holding my paper calendar in my hand hoping I can schedule them around my shows without coworkers noticing that something is up. I schedule like a pro.

I drive to my appointment with a sense of lightness. I already don a maxi pad and I know exactly what I am in for. I also think, well, I know I only had four follicles last time—so what, bring it!

This time my blood is drawn first. The nurse and I talk about movies. She wants to see *Despicable Me.*

I am called into the exam room by Unsexy Nurse Barbie. She is quite happy and leads me to the familiar setting. I feel comfortable and feel like nothing could go wrong—I have already experienced rock bottom, right?

She returns with a doctor I have not met, we introduce ourselves and the lights go dark and I take my position.

He slips it in and begins to count out loud, "One, two, three, four, five, six. Six on that side." "And, one, two, three on the other."

Nine! Nine follicles total! I am elated, smiling ear to ear—I can tell that the medical professionals are not happy but—nine! I had nine!

I return home filled with joy and tell Tim my news! They will call me that afternoon with results, but damn it, I increased my follicle count more than fifty percent!

I have the HSG a few days later. It takes place in their radiology department. It is much more clinical and cold there, also I discover that I am terrible at putting on hospital gowns. There are many snaps, ties and it seems there are too many arm holes. I stand there awkwardly for a few minutes trying to assess if they gave me incorrect garments. They give me two gowns and I am to wear them like a backwards robe, and the other like a normal robe. Easy, except I have the gowns that have not been snapped, but have been tied and washed too many times and the knots are impossible to get undone. I make my costume work and thankfully, I figure out the sock booties with no problems.

I am instructed to lie on an x-ray table, but in the gyno position. My doctor, a nurse and I wait for the x-ray technician to arrive. The doctor is in the ready position with a bulb syringe of dye to insert up my vagina, while the nurse will move the dentist-like x-ray device over my uterus and the x-ray tech (along with the rest of us) stare at the monitor to interpret the results. It is uncomfortable. It is weird and frankly, ancient—I ponder how far we have come as a society and yet, here we are about to shoot radioactive dye up my vag and watch it in real time flush my tubes.

We watch on the TV screen monitor the dye move up what looks like tree branches. Turns out, the uterus does not always look like what you learn in school—the triangle shape. Nope. My doctor starts telling me about all the weird shapes the uterus can be. Who knew? Apparently I passed this test.

Once the test is finished I had cramping and was leaking an iodine-looking substance for a few hours. I went to work, but I was cramped up for most of the day.

I get a call that my prolactin was still very high, follicle count was better—still not what they want to see, my FSH is still elevated and I have a very high antithyroglobulin. I am referred to an endocrinologist and I must make an appointment soon, the fertility team cannot continue.

They also got Tim's results. His motility was low; they now recommend in-vitro fertilization as our best course of action. However, I needed to see the endocrinologist before we can move forward.

In vitro fertilization is when fertilization of an egg takes place outside the body. In our case they were recommending IVF ICSI with assisted hatching. In vitro fertilization intracytoplasmic sperm injection. The process is what I like to think of as the bad-ass-hard core-fertilize-damn- it approach.

This is the process of IVF ICSI: after self injected medications manipulating my hormones to make as many follicles as I can (often call stimulation or stims), and daily monitoring of these follicles trans-vaginally at the fertility clinic, then at a specific time, I would get my final injected medication, a trigger shot, telling my body to ovulate. Thirty-five hours later I would be sedated and my doctor would, vaginally, insert a needle into my ovaries sucking out the fluid and follicles I had made. Once out, they would check to see which ones were viable. Then, in the lab my pretty, little follicles would have their outer shell removed (the assisted hatching part) and they would hand select the very best sperm Tim had offered. They would cut the tail off the sperm, and with a hollow needle—with the sperm head inside— stab it in to my follicle. They would do this as many times as there are viable follicles.

Depending on fertilization, between 3 and 5 days after the follicle retrieval, one or two embryos are then transferred vaginally into me, via a hmmm… I don't know what it looks like; let's say a turkey baster syringe. And hopefully, the embryo finds a cozy, sticky place to settle in for 38 or so weeks.

Why cut the tail off the sperm? (And when will you explain the nipple stimulation part?) Well, the tail's purpose in life is for movement, and in this case it would only cause destruction—so chop it off! The other form of IVF is that once the follicles are retrieved, they and the sperm hang out together in a dish the lab techs turn off the lights, put on some music and leave the room…

The why.

I am a triple threat. I used to joke that because I was blonde and Polish, I was a triple threat. I loved when people did not get the actual joke and tried to correct me that I had only named two things—people are funny…

But, I am a triple threat, at least when it comes to pregnancy. With my previous FSH tests I was told I was normal. I should have had someone explain that to me. When a patient has numbers in a normal range, the doctor usually then dismisses them as without issues. However, what may be normal for one woman may not be for another. In my circumstance, the fertility clinic's test was more in depth, looking for specific hormones and numbers.

Prolactin is the hormone the pituitary gland in your brain makes to motivate lactation—yup, breast milk. Remember the no nipple stimulation request? It is also the thread of truth to the old wives tale that a nursing woman cannot get pregnant—prolactin is nature's birth control. And, no, there was no milk leaking from my boobs…no milk…no big boobs…no infant… but I had sky high levels of prolactin.

On the first FSH my prolactin was the highest—as in twice the normal. They had me repeat the test fasting, and with *no nipple stimulation*. I had no idea what prolactin was and why in the world I had to re-do a blood test without eating and making out— it made no sense. Then I did a little research. The brain sends it out for a nursing mother to tell her body hey, not now, we are busy with an infant, and we cannot have another baby! Which is why it was assumed I must have been stimulating my nipples prior to the blood tests, how else could a non-lactating woman have this high of levels?

This began a series of tests; for every prolactin test, I was on the high end of the scale. Before every test I tell Tim that he can't even touch me! Thus begins our step one of getting pregnant—no sex.

Because of my high prolactin levels I am ordered to have an MRI of my brain. Prior to the MRI I was given a pregnancy test. (Let us pause, and soak that in…) I looked at the sample cup, the nurse, then the cup again. Sigh…you do realize why I have gathered you all here today, right? How optimistically cruel it is to hand a fertility patient a pee cup prior to an MRI. The MRI showed that I had a one millimeter adenoma (an adorable, cute, tumor) on my pituitary gland.

Next I learn that my antithyroglobulin antibodies were extremely high, as in four times the normal range. This is a marker for Hashimoto's disease, which means your body is attacking your thyroid. This can lead to a woman miscarrying. Which after reading all about this, Tim and I were not shocked to learn that there was a good possibility I had experienced miscarriages and did not know it.

Finally, point three of my triple threat; I have low ovarian function. At 31 my ovarian reserves were shockingly low, telling us that it is pretty soon that I will no longer be able to be in this child bearing race. This is the detail everyone seems to ignore. No one can comprehend this, they say *but you are so young, you have plenty of time, I had my kids at 47 after a bottle of Jameson and smoked a carton of Pall Malls a day.*

Hello, Jealousy, meet Rage.

Rage is who wanted to respond aloud to those who easily conceived… Oh, you lucky duck, what were your FSH levels at? What was your follicle count? Do you even know!? Did you cramp after your HSG? How many years did you try? How much did it cost you? You got pregnant. You prayed harder than me, you are nicer than me, prettier, smarter, richer, and more deserving—just say it, whatever you are trying to say, say it: You think that you are trying to motivate or support me? How does saying that you were older and in poor health and got pregnant support me? It does not. It infuriates me.

I am Rage. Another period will come and go. I wonder if that was my last follicle and there will be no more because we were too busy waiting on numbers and hormone levels.

There are no comforting words at any point in this race. It is silence, because when someone is silent it can be considered empathy, and that is all I want. I want someone to say, *what you are going through is terrible, I can't imagine your pain longing for a child.*

Endocrinology.

The endocrinologist I am referred to is no longer taking new patients and I will be seeing Dr. Pope instead. Hmm, Pope…seems like he'd be a nice guy.

The building, as I come to learn, will always have old crippled people hanging out in the lobby. I wonder if they are waiting for a shuttle. Old people sure do have a lot of appointments, then I wonder which doctor denomination are they there to see.

Dr. Pope's office is on the second floor. I prefer early appointments, simply because of traffic. The reception desks on the left are for endocrinology the ones on the right are for orthopedic surgeries and in the back is neurology. The endocrinology side is for the thyroid issues, like me, and those with diabetes.

Since I am a repeat patient they now smile at me and treat me a bit differently, but that first appointment, I felt like I was bad—like it was my fault I was there.

I pay my co pay and have a seat. I usually bring my coffee and sip quietly in the back. I smile at the others waiting and notice that I am much younger and feel so small.

I am called in and my weight is checked. I don't remove my shoes. I am not sure why. In some way, maybe it is pride—or trying to show that I don't care. But I do, I look to see what it says. Then she asks me the standard questions: did he give you any medications, did you get lab work done, and where? Then she takes my pulse and blood pressure.

I am fiercely proud of my pulse. Becoming a runner has made my pulse in the low sixty's, sometimes even the fifty's. Whenever someone in the medical profession takes my pulse they ask me if I am a runner and tell me, they knew because my pulse was so low. I take it as a compliment, proof that I am athletic and healthy—regardless that I now have an endocrinologist and can't get pregnant.

They never check my blood pressure using the wall-mount gauges, always the rolling nomad machine. Are the ones on the wall, props, like TGI Fridays décor?

The rooms are old. They have the patient table with the butcher paper, but it feels unsanitary. There are two chairs and the rolling stool. I always sit in the chair, clearly the rolling stool is for the doctor and the table is only if for some reason I needed a physical exam.

There is a drawer labeled *vaginal speculums*. I question this in my head. Is this a rummage sale table and they could not peel the label off? There are no stirrups on the table. Whose bright idea was it that gynecological exam tables needed stirrups? Why not make the table wider but with foot gutters on the sides? Some dude's sick, horse fantasy probably. And while we are at it, who do we need to petition for gently warmed, silicone speculums? The technology exists…can we get on this, please?

Dr. Pope becomes one of my favorite doctors throughout my baby quest. He is socially awkward, young and speaks as though I am an informed individual. We will see each other many times in the upcoming year, as I am put on thyroid medication and he calculates my dosage as my blood work is done every 4 weeks. Turns out the numbers on my blood panel should be at a certain level for fertility—though this is not the case for every woman; he does a mathematical formula and prescribes the dosages. (Interesting how this magic fertility number never came up before with any other doctor.) He asks routine questions of me: have I been getting headaches, how is my vision, (a pituitary adenoma can cause headaches and changes in vision) he checks my weight and asks me how my marathon training is going (the thyroid issue that threatens me is one that its symptoms are lethargy and weight gain). He also checks my reflexes, and my arms to see if the medication is causing any tremors. Our visits are quick. But in these short visits I learn a lot about the thyroid. It is a terribly important gland; if not balanced you can be hyperthyroidism or hypothyroidism. My tests are showing that I may be hypo in the future, but not now. Currently what we are trying to mitigate is the Hashimoto's, which is something I will always have, but not always need medication for.

He also informs me that there is not a lot of data he can consult about my particular situation. It's not a gamble to put me on the thyroid medication, in fact with Hashimoto's it is necessary to be on thyroid medicine prior to getting pregnant since in the first trimester the baby depends on the mother's thyroid. Since my body is attacking my thyroid…well you see why the medication is needed…The humorous detail is that there is an ethical issue of women being on thyroid medication during pregnancy—apparently there is data that those babies have higher IQ's. Great, go through all this and my baby is going to be a genius—crap!

Betrayed by my body.

I was taught if you work hard, apply yourself and do your very best, you can achieve anything. If you want a high paying job, you get the right schooling and training, get the interview and you can get the job. If you want a certain house, you save the money, be smart about your budgets, spending and credit, you can get that house. I was taught that menstruation was one of the key components towards motherhood. I was taught to wait. I was taught to expect that one day, I would be pregnant. I had the hardware, I had the tools, the plans, and it was time.

This diagnosis of infertility became such a betrayal, a harsh smack of reality. I will not get what I want, the way that I want it. Jealousy, Rage, meet Selfish… My body, my strong, sleek and cute body was not able to produce the results that I wanted through trying, studying, or luck. I needed help, medical help. I sunk into shame. The major, natural thing a woman can do, the thing that every month for years my body had systematically done for 5 to 7 days, was a sham. A lie. I could not have a baby. I could not get pregnant.

Jealousy, negative, hate and tears.

When you start trying to conceive everyone in your orbit will be pregnant. It is a fact, women will either be announcing they are pregnant or visibly pregnant, it will even feel like all the men in your life are with child too. When you want something so bad, I find that there is always that one person who has what you want and they become not a beacon of hope-but the bane of your existence. Someone who you just cannot believe they are so fortunate. That snake of jealousy is called up from its cozy coil in your stomach, rhythmically being sung up to the top of your skull as they charm their way through their perfect life. Perfect everything. I realize how truly long I had wanted a baby as I indulge self pity and recount journal entries.

December 19, 2009

We are not/will not be pregnant in 2009. Of course I am sad and a bit depressed. But it is okay. What is happening now is there is a blizzard warning. We already have snow on the ground and it is supposed to keep falling all day...

November 12, 2010

This morning I prayed an entire rosary so that I may move through my jealous state. I admitted to God that the only way I would know if I have learned this step and came through it, is to be tested. To hear about someone's pregnancy and feel joy for them.

I viewed a friends' home video of his new son learning to crawl. I cried, a short cry, but one of sheer longing. Clearly, I am not there yet.

It is shameful to admit, but there is one mother whose good fortune sent me into a furious spiral. The madness when your body tingles with pain, like pins and needles when seated too long, but without the sympathy of others as you stomp around the

room wailing that your foot fell asleep. It is an unbearable ache
and sends me into tears so easily.

She got married and, well, damn near close to that day, she
conceived. She called us within a few weeks of her finding out
and it sent me into a fit of tears, jealous tears. Tim and I fought
that night. This was about two years prior to us seeking the
fertility clinic; Tim told me we were not pregnant because we
were not consistent and we were not doing everything possible to
get pregnant and that we should be happy for her. Just like a
man, we aren't having enough sex….
What he didn't know was that I was upset because at her wedding
reception she told me and her mother that she and I were *racing
to get pregnant*. Her news upset me, because I knew in my heart
there was something wrong with us, and that yet again, she got
what she wanted and I did not.

I was asked to take part in the planning of the baby shower and I
was deeply hurt. I was hurt that no one realized that it may be
awkward for me to help put on a baby shower. They knew we
were trying and it seems they quickly had forgotten.

About a week before her baby shower, I was incredibly stressed
with work and the anxiety of seeing her pregnant pushed me over
the edge, well, actually it pushed me to crumple on our kitchen
floor in a heap of tears. I admitted to Tim that I did not want to
go to her shower. He called her mom for me and let her know
that I had the *flu*. We then fought.

We saw them at Christmas, she was due at any moment, and it
took every ounce of courage I had to see her, to be loving and
kind. I judged everything. What she was eating, how she looked,
how she complained, how the house looked—I judged like the
mean and ungrateful woman that I am. And I saw my own
hideous self, and hated me even more. No wonder I could not
conceive, I was filled with hate.

I have heard that sometimes God will bless someone else just to see how you react. Though I did not outwardly express it, I felt mean, full to the brim hate filled mean. I wanted her to hurt. I wanted everyone to hurt.

When she was in labor, I judged some more. I could not be genuinely excited or happy for her. Her blessing caused me so much misery.

Her son was the first grandchild in her family. There are many pictures and visits to see his first fill-in-the-blank holiday. I am an aunt twenty-one times. When Tim married me, he was an automatic uncle.

For some reason, it was her pregnancy that filled me with jealousy. It almost made me feel like I will never have this—like she was the last woman on Earth God was going to allow being pregnant, and I lost. For every other pregnancy, I didn't have that ache, with everyone else, I actually had hope. Maybe because they are directly related to me by a sibling—which yes, logically makes no sense—but go with it…

So now, with another holiday season approaching, with my heart heavy, how do you move through this? How, do you see yourself as such a hate-filled, sad, pathetic, barren woman and wish your family and friends a Merry Christmas and talk to your nieces about Santa and Barbie? To not be happy for someone with their joy, is a dark, dank, smelly place.

Jealousy, Rage, Selfishness meet Self Loathing.

November 27, 2010

So, she is pregnant again.

I went into our family room, curled up on the couch with our dog and watched some Springsteen, a concert I have on our DVR.
Oh, and I cried.

I am jealous. I am mad. I hate myself. I am supposed to be the one getting pregnant. I am supposed to be one day closer. But I am currently in limbo with my period waiting for my case nurse to tell me to start the birth control pills, but it is Thanksgiving and my uterus' timing is remarkably evil. How did I get the evil uterus? I am kind. I mean, I am really kind; I donate to charities, both monetarily and otherwise. In fact, there is a bag of clothing in my foyer waiting for me to call for its pick-up. I go to church. I listen to my students and I encourage them to be better. I am so polite in traffic. I smile at people. I am generous, when people come over our house they never leave hungry or thirsty. I do the runners nod at every one I see while running. We are nice people. Why does getting pregnant have to be so damn hard?

It is not about being kind. Or luck. Or favor. My life has a path. I think I know where it is going, but that is a load of crap. I have no idea. There was a time I thought I did; there was a time where I could not understand why any woman would want to give up their job and stay at home to be a mom. There was a time that my job was my identity. The reality is, that time was not too long ago. Infertility and the news of my own body's inability to perform its primary function in my gender, made me seek my identity. It made me seek God, the wonder and beauty in the world around me. I saw that I was bigger than my job. I impacted people, no matter my vocation. In a supermarket or a doctor's office, I could make someone's day. I could choose to be the positive customer; I could be the one who lets you in at the merge. It doesn't matter how much I make, but what I am made of.

For all of this I had to seek God, but I don't think She is for everyone. Tim is an atheist and that works for him, and oddly enough, it works for me. We actually respect each other's opinions. He worries that making it to church stresses me out— so I make sure that it doesn't. Yes, I think God is a She and I think She has a plan for me, and I truly believe She has not left me alone during all of this. She may have helped *her* get pregnant just to see how I would take it. The jury is still out as to whether or not I passed. Her timing is not mine, but I think I need to do everything possible, and do all that I can, and leave the rest to Her.

While praying, I told God that I was mad she was pregnant, because she was such a brat. I felt Her response as, *brats get pregnant too.*

Who am I to judge who gets to get pregnant? Is there a requirement? Certainly there is not a height, weight, age, race criteria. If there was, I certainly would not be in the predicament I am now, I am a 5'-4" 135 pound 31 year old white woman, I am as average and boring as anyone you got!

So, why me?

That is a stupid question.

Because, no one can go through this quite like me. I am average and healthy, someone you would not expect with infertility. I am happily married and fortunately this has not affected the marriage. I am strong and determined, calculated and spontaneous. I like tequila, I have Celiac disease and I love my cankles. I got big plans to be a mom, and I am currently ironing out the kinks in the details.

So, she is pregnant. So fucking what? No, I am not in the place to be able to happily call with congratulations and squeal with delight. I am not in the place to get excited about baby clothes, gifts and a baby shower. For the time being, I need to step back. To sit with grace and journal it out, so that maybe one day, I can share it and help someone who at that time, is in that place of silently sighing, *it is not fair.* And, no, it is not fair.

With each day, I am one day closer.

I am a jealous person. I know this. I mean I really know this—I sit in it. I am seeking to find the reason we are traveling through this, and so far the only thing I can really think of is that I need to get over myself and mind my own business. I can't be the first infertile woman who is jealous of others pregnancies. How do they do it? Or are they fake, hiding and secretly mourning, like me.

I want to get to that place of joy for others. I think that hope is a big part of it. I want to think that re-telling my sad story will help, but it won't. Well, not me at least. Re-hashing this with the intentions of getting sympathy or so someone will shut up about their baby joy…that is not who I want to be.

Being social or living in the age of social networking is not the friend of infertility. It is every day that someone is either announcing their pregnancy, complaining about their burgeoning belly, counting the days until their delivery or talking about being a mom.

How do I show them love? Currently, I ignore any post. Currently, I am anxious before any family gathering fearing that someone will ask me when we are going to have a baby, which, I might add, is the worst, most offensive thing you can say to a woman. Some think it is the *C* word—I beg to differ, someone who calls me that is clearly mad at me and is expressing themselves—good for them. Someone who is asking about a private matter is an ignorant sloth. (That was not a very loving way to deal with my emotions…) No one asks men, *how is your penis? Have you had your semen analyzed—cause, you know, you really should have knocked her up by now!*

I have been judgmental. I have very easily offended many people and chalked it up to being blunt or having a sense of humor. Sadly, I don't know who to apologize to, and I am not sure for what. But I see it now.

I am hoping that through all of this I will be a better person. No, in fact, I want to be awesome. I want to be the spokesperson for getting through life's shit with a grace that lights up a room! I am scared though. And, I understand why pregnant woman talk so much about their condition. They are scared too. There are so many unknowns and things that can happen. They have to give over their entire body to another being, nourish it, love it, and when it comes out, it is her priority forever. But, there are books about it. And many other woman who have been through it whom are happy to advise, hell, they will even strike up conversations in the grocery store with a woman who is expecting—unsolicited stranger advice! But this, infertility, is a sad and lonely struggle. Only other infertile women know what this is like—and I haven't met them; there are no widely marketed support groups, meetings or clubs. I am too ashamed to start one.

Tim finally told his family, but no one called or checked in to see how I was holding up. I guess that confirms that I really want sympathy, maybe empathy. I don't want to be alone in this mess. I want them to choose their words more carefully. I want apologies. I want acknowledgment that they do not understand, and cannot imagine the devastation of this and want to know how they can help or support us. I want to be surrounded by love. But, it will never be enough. I am in a state where I cannot get what I want when I want it—and I despise others who have what I want. What kind of terrible person am I?

 Sad part is, the truly sad part is, that I know that this stress and negativity is the opposite of what I need. I know that I need to manage my stress, my anger and my jealousy. I know that I need to think of speedy sperm, expectant follicles, happy fat babies cooing and spit up, full breasts and diaper bags...but when I see a mom...I see a woman who is better than me, because she can conceive. My insecurity is so palatable that I swell with jealousy at her sight. I know I am supposed to learn something from every hardship in life. I wish I was a fast learner... I think this is telling me how selfish I am and can be. How my feelings rule my thoughts and actions—and how much I am actually not in control. That, is a very difficult realization. That is why I have been angry for so long, how nothing is good enough, no one can do anything right. How is it possible to let go of all of that while struggling to pursue getting what you want?

Can I love others through this? Can I be authentically joyful when others conceive?

Holidays suck. Gatherings of any sort with even one couple that has a child, is torture. Everyone talks about the funny/cute/smart child. And parents, once they become parents they have nothing else to talk about but being parents and those without children are nothing and know nothing of the world at all, because they are not a parent.

Apparently, when you become a parent is the only time one understands and knows the concept of tired, and everything else in the world. I get it; you don't sleep when you have a child—ever.

Also, being a parent entitles you to be an asshole. This also includes those expecting to be parents. They are experts on how to get pregnant, being pregnant, and how to be the best human being in the world. They know everything and are happy to impart their wisdom to you whether or not you asked. For, just being in their presence means that you wish to have some slice of their knowledge.

I am amazed at the audacity parents have. It is not uncommon for someone to touch a woman's pregnant belly, without her permission! How is this okay? I think I would slap their hand down and shout, *No! Bad!*

Joining the infertility club has taught me many things. Holiday cards with photos of children, happy families, pregnant women or sonogram photos are pompous and arrogant. Before our diagnosis, I was convinced that we would do something cute like those photo cards; in fact I was looking forward to it. But in our current state, when we receive those cards, I open them, glance, and my body cringes. I begin to feel angry and sad. It is a weird depression; others joy brings about such an angry power surge, like I am the Incredible Hulk, complete with the ripped clothing and green skin.

Hmm, green with envy. The green-eyed monster. I wonder if Hulk had infertility. It explains everything; who would procreate with a man who gets that angry and wears frayed, cut off jean shorts?

In fact most any baby related thing provokes the jealous monster in me. Seeing photos, toys, and baby cups—items which should be in any grandmother's house, but to me, it is a cruel reminder.

It is as if the world does revolve around me. How dare they not realize my sensitive state! And it is equally cruel that you can buy these baby items in general grocery stores, gas stations, bars, arcades. Can I not escape it?!

 Is my jealousy so rampant because my hope is currently in the hands of God's timing and a team of doctors? Did the knowledge of what was wrong with our bodies cause me to be more jealous, angrier? I remember being sad, I remember crying at every menstrual period—but I had a glimmer of hope, now what I have is still hope, but it does not glimmer. It is a reality of hope. There is no sparkly shimmer dust, it is like I know completely how hard this will be, and yet I am still doing it. It is filthy hope. It is elbow grease hope. Maybe it is a gift, to go through this. Fertile woman get thrown into pregnancy, there is immediate joy and wonder, then a sense of miracles taking place every day, then they are showered with gifts and strangers telling them how glow-y they are, then the pain of labor and delivery and bam, crying, sleeplessness and the journey of the unexpected begins.

Whereas, my whole journey starts with the unexpected, I get to go through an immense path of questions, the dark unknown, and the elbow grease style work, complete dependency on others, asking for help, learning grace, learning patience, learning and experiencing that I will not get what I want, when I want it. Then, God willing, then I experience the wonder, joy and miracle, and I will embrace it fully, because I will have been in absolute darkness and each day forward is bright and more brilliant than where I have been.

Yeah, that makes me feel better.

People talk about babies a lot. But the conversation is never about how hard it is to conceive or infertility. It is always about happy unplanned or planned pregnancies; it is almost nonchalant. Like noticing someone's new haircut. Even when someone purchases a new home it is a surprise achievement. How come when someone is pregnant we assume it was super easy for them? Was it? Is it? Are we so ignorant to the subject of infertility that we can't be amazed that a man and a woman came together at precisely the right time, with precisely the right circumstances and hormones and health factors to create another living being! Are we too jaded to see the miracle in that?

I certainly was. Still am, when it comes to others. For me, this wonderment is out of reach, and I will need to do everything possible to have it, but until someone tells me otherwise, I am the only infertile woman I know.

The miracle of life gives pregnant ladies a *glow*. I wonder if when I am pregnant I will glow. Or am I jaded? Or, can I be eternally in awe that life provided me such an opportunity?

It seems to me, that there is a constant battle for my attention. To engage in the anger, jealousy and the wicked thoughts towards those I deem lucky *or* to embrace the hope that one day I will be lucky too. The healthier version, of course is to embrace. To feel blessed, to enjoy the day and the moment. It does not always work, and there seems to be a moment, if not several, out of each day that I engage the beast. But, then I take a deep breath, and I think of the happiest place I have been, or maybe some of my happiest moments and I allow my mind and spirit to go there. I recount the weather, the sounds, the feeling on my skin… Often, I can open my eyes and begin anew. I can forgive myself for having thoughts of rage, I can forgive others for whatever I think they may have done or said. I can be calm and see life for what it is: perfect. Everything is perfect, in its own way—what I think has no bearing on its perfection. I too am perfect, though I may not see how yet, I will.

This is only a test.

Roller Girl.

I rush to the clinic for a fluid sonogram and mock embryo transfer; these are the next tests on the list towards IVF. I am happy that they do a practice run for a transfer, instead of figuring it out when they are trying to implant my precious cargo.

I read the information pamphlet and dangers the night before at our dining room table. I was spread out, with medical notes, my notebooks and concern wiped all over my face. (PRO TIP: get a notebook and a folder or binder to keep all your information straight; the clinic will provide information but usually it is generic to the procedure, and chances are your protocol is going to be a cacophony of large words, schedules and a specific medicine regimen, you need to put on your Type A pants to *handle* infertility…and your Type B pants on to *live* with infertility.) The fluid sonogram sounds like a terrible procedure. Test after test sounds unpleasant. For this one, they will insert a vaginal speculum—or metal duckbill, clean me with surgical soap and then proceed to fill my uterus with saline and take a vaginal ultrasound. They are looking for fibroids or anything that will get in the way of a baby. After that is done, they will do the mock transfer, in which they map out and measure how they will do the eventual transfer of a fertilized embryo in me, like an embryo dress rehearsal.

I arrive at the office, am ushered into a patient room and I undress from the waist down; I am getting very used to this process. I am so comfortable getting undressed from the waist down I am surprised this hasn't translated to other public activities I engage in whenever my name is called…*Venti latte for Mary! Walk up, drop my jeans, hop on the counter fold a napkin on my lap and wait.* I am in the same room I was the last time I was here. There is very little reading material on the wall. It is clean. I leave my socks on, and I hope that it will not take too long. I think about work, and what I need to do there and I wish that Tim were with me.

The Physician's Assistant and a nurse come in. Both are gorgeous women, blonde and happy. Fertile, probably.

I joke that this sounds like a horrible test; she assuages my fears and tells me that it actually takes longer to read the consent forms then it does to perform the procedure. She is right.

I felt some pain and cramping—but not much else.

While she was doing the mock transfer I heard her say,

"Oooh, hmmm... your cervix is a bit tricky. It goes back, and then to the right..." "Okay, you are done, but don't sit up yet—take a moment and get up slowly."

"Is everything normal?" I ask.

"Oh, yes, I mapped it out, the technician will have my notes, once you are in, it will be just fine."

She tells me that it was nice to meet me, and she exits. The nurse gives me a wipe, a comically giant maxi pad and paperwork to hand in at the front desk. I am told to have a nice day and given some privacy to wipe and get dressed. I feel wet and cramped. I feel like I have been menstruating for weeks with all the tests and vaginal ultrasounds it is simply easier to use pads and I hate pads so much.

I leave the clinic feeling okay—like I accomplished something. They now have notes as to how to get my fertilized egg back into my body—that is good, right? I get into the car and head to work.

If I ever become a roller derby girl, I have my name: *Tricky Cervix*.

Tricky Cervix soon becomes the manifestation of the woman I want to be. An alter ego. *Tricky* is not only a roller girl (which I have no tangible experience with) but she is a bad ass mom. She is physically strong, her body slender and scarred with epic stories of roller derby bouts and life. Her hair is tinged with lavender, because she doesn't care, she is pierced and tattooed and all the while earthy, hippy and kind. She always has time for friends, family and work. She is balanced and happy while giving away nothing that she doesn't want to give. She is the one you call to vent, she is the one you call for a solution and the one you call so her light can cast down on your dark existence helping you find your way back. She does yoga, roller derby, marathons, rock climbing and can knit. She grows her own food, has chickens and is never alone unless she asks for it. She is beautiful, naturally but can create the perfect smoky eye and her nails are always painted. She welds and can hot wire cars. She laughs without hesitation and can make friends with a zombie. She is in perfect balance with the spirit and physical world. She is fertile but isn't a jerk about it. I find parts of her attainable, hell parts that I already have, yet all the while I find that the woman I am is lacking—suffering—instead of understanding impermanence, acceptance and balance. Finding who I want to be is in part the act of reinventing myself, and this desire towards motherhood is just that. I don't want to be the fun aunt, but I need to figure out how to be happy being the fun aunt if that is what is to be. I need to harness my *Tricky Cervix*.

Patience.

I cannot help but wonder if I must go through this for some reason, some purpose, and preparation for what is to come. Is this training or teaching me for the hardship I will endure? What if our baby will have a disability that will require all of my attention and patience; will this long test be what is required for me to parent him or her? I feel the need to have a reason for this. I feel that this is my moment, each day, to get through this with grace and peace. To learn to be loving, kind and happy with where I am today.

I have heard sermons that patience is not about waiting for what you want, but how you act while you are waiting. When women all around you are announcing pregnancies and dropping out babies, how do you smile gracefully, how do you find peace knowing that you will not have their easy road? In what do you find enjoyment during the hard moments?

I start doing more yoga, I don't have a teacher or studio, I read about what poses are good for fertility and health and I try and mimic them. I start visualizing being a mom, thinking about my *Tricky Cervix* qualities I want to hone and how to move forward. There is a lot of emphasis placed on trying yoga or acupuncture for infertility. Because, you know what is some more needles? Fundamentally, it makes sense. Balance…moderation, bad days, good days. The calming breath work and stretching makes me feel physically good, but I find my mat wet with tears most days. I feel alone.

I keep a journal, I make New Year's goals, I track good things, bad things, random things; this is how I stay in balance best. Usually after venting into a notebook either I come up with a solution, or I realize what my next steps should be. Usually journaling is great, except when you look back and realize how long you have been trying to have a baby. That is a lot of zero return sex.

July 27, 2006

Tomorrow I am off birth control. I need to make a gyno appointment. In the meantime Tim is up for a baby if that is meant to be.

July 30, 2006

Today, Tim and I had total unprotected sex. Not with the sole intention of getting pregnant, but we welcome the possibility.

January 1, 2007

Health

Happiness

A license to drive

January 1, 2008

The thought of purchasing a home has crept into our heads; they are raising the rent of our apartment... we will be headed out to look at homes in what may be our price range. We do not have a realtor, just an estimate loan number given to us by the bank. I am applying for the manager job in my department, and my skin is horribly breaking out. I have my period, so that does not help. I have a lot on my plate, and maybe a new home will kick start my ambition to getting my license and relax me for conceiving— maybe that is my problem. I am so damn anxious!

December 24, 2008

Together we bought a Led Zeppelin onesie for the baby we do not yet have.

[Hindsight: I am so glad we went for a classic band rather than something short lived like Milli Vanilli.] *The year is almost to an end, so much wonderfulness has happened, at times it is like life re-began when grandma died. She is helping us. We are in a wonderful, safe new home with life ahead of us. All I need surrounds me, I simply need to accept it.*

January 7, 2009

I rang in the New Year with a bad cold. I am giving myself permission to stay home sick. Tim came home early from work today. I know that in time we will get pregnant, and it is okay. We are where we need to be in our lives right now. I can give more to others, I can be more forgiving, I can practice both patience and letting go, and I can find peace with surrendering.

December 19, 2009

We are not/will not be pregnant in 2009. Of course I am upset, sad and a bit depressed. But it is okay.

January 1, 2010

Resolutions:

To teach yoga

To run a marathon

To be a mother

To be debt free

To know God

To engage in charity work

To find the happiness inside of me

December 31, 2010

We will not be pregnant in 2010. But, we know why. I have had miscarriages we believe, many tests, and now a plan for IVF ICSI. We have a team of doctors and a have the support of my family and friends. I have a sister in law who has been through it and will support me every step of the way. Tim is my solid strength, I am loved. Though I am not getting what I want, when I want it...yet, I smile!

January 1, 2011

2010 was a year of learning.

I learned about my physical self; my infertility, health issues and that I can push myself and run a marathon.

I learned about my spiritual self; I began a faithfulness journey of prayer, learning the role God is in my life and that joy and happiness comes from within.

I learned about my emotional self, how strong feelings of anger and jealousy emerge quickly, how to be brave and move forward afraid. How to seek peace and ask for help.

My resolution for 2011 is simple and complex: to grow.

I resolve to grow physically with a baby, to do all the necessary things for my health—to pay attention to my body.

I resolve to grow spiritually with God, to grow a closer relationship with Her.

I resolve to grow emotionally, to move through with grace, to be brave and kind, to pause before reacting, to be patient, kind, compassionate and loving to all—to grow up.

Running with God.

On October 16th, 2010 I ran in the Baltimore Running Festival. Specifically, the Under Armor Baltimore Marathon. 26.2 miles in the slowest time ever, I wasn't last, but I wasn't fast.

I trained for a year, the previous year I ran the half marathon and while running it, I thought, *I will run the full marathon next year.* And, I did. How fitting for this to be the year I train for a marathon and also learn of my infertility. It is not a sprint…blah, blah, blah worst cliché ever…

My race was painful and lonely.

I did not have a running buddy and the pace group I anticipated running with, well, I lost them soon after the start. I had myself. So, I prayed. At each mile marker I said a Hail Mary, when I hit ten I said an Our Father, then for the next decade I did two Hail Mary's at every mile. It was like the marathoners version of the rosary.

At every mile I hoped that next year at this time, I will be training to deliver a baby or babies.

I do not have a cathartic description of crossing the finish line. I did my very best for that day. I accepted myself and my circumstances. In my head I plan to run one every year—hoping, God willing, I can take off one year to be pregnant and deliver a healthy baby.

There are not many people who can say they have run a marathon. In fact, they say that if you can run a marathon, there is not a whole lot you can't do.

There are also not many people who have been able to say to me that they understand what Tim and I are going through. We are in the club, and there are times I wish we were not.

To train for a marathon you need few things. Good sneakers, time to train and discipline. I guess determination fits in there too—but if you signed up for a marathon, determination is a part of the registration fee. What I also needed, though, was support and information. I read websites and magazines about running, and my husband—mister sports fan, was easy to rope in as my support crew. Time was difficult, my work hours were never normal, and when I was home there were chores to be done and food to prepare. But oddly enough, my sister texted me one day asking if I wanted her treadmill, and if I could trade her, our crock pot. To me, this was such an incredible gift!

The room that got the treadmill was our dreamy expected nursery. We had painted it *Orange Blast*, soon after we moved in. It reminded me of a creamsicle.

Most days, I would run in our nursery to be. During my training, we thought it could be at any month we would be pregnant; I would have to defer the marathon, plans would change and oh, how wonderful! But each month approached, and the nursery stayed orange blast, stayed crib-less. We soon began to call it the exercise room, and we did not dare tour guests the house and call that room the nursery—too many questions and expectations. I could not admit what failures we were.

I have many Dr. Seuss books. Weird story. When I was about twelve I signed up for a book club, a Dr. Seuss book club, kind of like those one cent CD clubs. In fact, exactly like a one cent CD club. My plan was that I would then have all of these great Dr. Seuss books for my future children. I still have them, every once in a while when we need a child's gift in a pinch I take one from the pile, but I still have plenty. Twelve year old Mary never imagined it would be a trial to get a baby, obviously, she thought the biggest problem was that the world would stop printing Dr. Seuss books, and so she had to stockpile them.

I would run, look at the room, books, the paint I chose and would intensely imagine the crib, the changing table, the rocking chair, the drapes. We needed better drapes, there is no way anyone could have a successful nap with those drapes!

I would imagine the day we found out. I day dreamed our baby shower. What my smile would look like? What pregnant Mary would look like? Would she run? Would our baby run? What would they become in this crazy world? I imagine all of this so intently that it feels real, and that only heightens the pain. It is walking the line of seeing the positive possibilities and not getting overwhelmed in the sheer reality of negative nothingness.

I started taking God seriously after we learned about my diagnosis. Oddly enough, some of my 2010 resolutions are as follows:

Run a marathon

Become a mom/get pregnant

Know God

Practice patience

The last two, I admit, I had no idea what they meant. To me, at the time, running a marathon and getting pregnant were easy list items I could cross off. I actually had them on a list—who does that?

But, practicing patience and knowing God? I was not enthusiastic about how to do those. I don't even know what I was going after when I added them. I guess they were in my heart, things that I deeply wanted but not the *thinking Mary*, the Mary that has feelings and vibes and mothers others without knowing— the *spiritual Mary* wanted them on her list.

I started going to church, mainly because I was asked to be a godmother and needed to register at a church. The baptism was on August 8th, 2010. It was August 9th, 2010 I was given the news that my test results for fertility were *not encouraging*. I went to church to hear something. To hear divine news. To get a revelation about my life and how to make it better. I wanted action steps for my check list. There were some Sundays that I did indeed enjoy the homily and get something out of it. It is not a chore for me, but it has become something of an appointment to keep with myself. I started to ponder my work schedule, could I somehow ensure that I would get mass time off? If orthodox Jews can make it work, why can't I?

I also started really praying. I pray the rosary. I have prayed for my enemies—which oddly enough include all pregnant women—and anyone who annoys me. I have prayed for mine and all women's fertility and I have prayed that God would not forget me. As if there are a certain number of pregnancies allotted and a prayer would remind God I wanted in on the list. I have prayed for forgiveness, and felt—well, forgive yourself. It is hard not to feel that this infertility is a punishment. But it is not; I cannot think that. I have to believe that it means something, that it will mean something.

I believe the Hail Mary is the prayer for the infertile woman. At least, after saying it every day now for a while (I have no sense of time) I had a revelation that this was the prayer for me. One woman, asking another woman, to pray for her, for she had what the other wanted and maybe, just maybe her grace could intercede for the woman desiring a child. Worth a shot, right?

And, so I pray. Sometimes I have feeling behind it, sometimes I get lost in thought. But for a brief period of my day I feel like I am making progress. I pray while I run, I create a habit of it.

I imagine God running with me. More like Jesus running with me, He looks like the pictures of typical Jesus with a sad face the looking off into the distance; however I imagine Him in a white tank top, sometimes t-shirt, shorts and a sweatband on his forehead. For some reason, running Jesus in my head is stuck in the 1980's with *way* too short of shorts. Also, I am always ahead of Him, like I need to look back to see if He is still with me. How's that metaphor for you?

Maybe I need to strive for the image of Jesus running side by side with me. I will pray for that. So now I run with Jesus and have

this alter ego roller girl? I think instead of baby fever, I may have
a mental illness going on.

Acceptance.

I have accepted that my body, in its current state, in union with Tim's body and his current state, will not create a baby without the help of science. It has taken a long time. Daily I think, positively, believing that a baby will come into my life somehow, someway…

I have moved passed accepting. I expect it now. I expect that we will very soon begin the process of in vitro fertilization. I expect that I will diligently take my pills, injections and suppositories. I will get my blood drawn, I will follow my calendar of appointments, and I expect that we will be successful and that within our three attempts that our insurance allows, we will become pregnant. I expect that I will carry my baby a full term and deliver a healthy baby or two, or three or four… I expect days that I will pity myself and cry for too long. I expect stress and doubt. I expect to be expecting. I actually say this to myself daily: a baby will come into my life somehow, someway.

November 11, 2010

We have the green light! Dr. Pope has given us (the fertility team) the go ahead!

Though my prolactin was still high, he says it is in the normal range, and my TSH is where we need it, below 2.5. All of the hormones secreted by the pituitary gland were normal, so Dr. Pope has given us the go ahead to start the in-vitro process.

I am feeling proud of my body, like I accomplished something!

I tell Tim, and he seems so excited. I have forgotten that he has been a patient through this too; he has had to wait and cannot do anything about it. I have to take the medicine, I have to schedule and maintain blood work and get things straight. He must feel helpless—I haven't even bothered to ask.

We now wait some more. On day one of my next period I call
our case nurse and from there we start birth control pills then the
injections. I do hope that in the meantime we can get pregnant on
our own. It would be funny and, well, easier. I do not wish this
on anyone.

November 12, 2010

*I want this experience. I want in vitro to work. I want multiples,
mainly because I want more than one child and I fear this is our
only shot. I want to write this book. I want it to help other
women get through this dark hole.*

I want this to be the greatest lesson of my life. I want to recount
and learn from each day I obsess over it. I want my children to
understand, to know, how much they meant to me before they
were even conceived.

Any fool can have sex and get pregnant. But it takes a
committed, loving, strong, faith-filled woman to willingly go
through the path of in vitro fertilization or any other fertility
treatment.

December 12, 2010
*What is upcoming? In 2011 we will journey deeper into IVF.
With appointments, injections, medications, stress and tests; there
is a lot for us to tackle.*

I am scared.

*I can work myself up into a frenzy wondering if it will work, if we
will be okay, if we can handle it--if I can handle it. If this
transaction is blessed. Is God on our side with this--is this truly
how it is supposed to go? Would I be able to get pregnant if I did
not have this craptastic job that steals my joy and spirit? But,
this job's insurance is paying for this. How does one go through
this without insurance? What is my purpose for going through
this—how can I make this so exceedingly helpful to someone else
to balance out this pain?*

Every year, I expect us to get pregnant, I fear disappointment. What if this does not work?

I don't want my story to be of the infertile woman. But I want everyone else to hurt as much as I do. How unfair is that—is that what normal people feel like?
A student asked me, *when are you going to have kids*? I simply replied that it was none of her business. I wonder what it takes for people to realize how painful their innocent questions truly are.

December 27, 2010

I am researching pharmacies. You do not get IVF drugs at the CVS around the corner. This is a pain. I was given three brochures, told they were all great and now I have to make a decision. One is local—which would be our number one choice, but they do not have a good website nor someone on call 24 hours a day—which given the situation, I feel is necessary. The other two are a toss-up, one in NJ-my home state, but their site is not very informative and way more on the pictures of babies, sentimental side. The other is in Massachusetts as well as Rhode Island. I am uneasy as to how often we will need emergency delivery of medication. After all, we are new to this, and to be frank, I do not want to be a repeat customer. Basically, I am deciding whom I want to have my insurance and my money, and whom will I hold accountable when shit goes wrong. I wish CVS did do fertility drugs, and did have a 24/7 service. Why has this not happened? Do you know how much this stuff costs? Ridiculous.

It is also ridiculous that I have to pay to do something so many can do naturally. I don't want to be angry (such a common theme) but it really is difficult. How do you overcome the anger? How in the world do you move through this?

With God? Is God the answer? How are you supposed to get through this? Spoiler alert, no one has ever answered this simple question.

December 28, 2010

I started my second pack of birth control pills today, this is still baffling to me, but they want to control all of my hormones, and this is the way to do it. Because of spotting it was as if I had my period twice in a month. What a treasure that was. Way to stick the knife in deeper, fertility clinic! Anyway, it would be super awesome if that was my last period for a while…

The plan is that I take this pack of active pills and straight into a third pack, we return from vacation on January 17th, and on the 18th I have an ultrasound and blood work. This will be much like my FSH tests, I expect, and with this I am hoping for more of a concrete calendar of events.

I asked my nurse to fax over my prescription list to the pharmacy we have decided to use.   I chose the local one. My specific questions were as follows:

Do you take my pharmacy insurance?

Do you take major credit cards?

Do you keep my medications on site—then I listed them.

What happens if I have an emergency need after your hours of operation?

She answered all to my satisfaction, and so they win my money, and insurance claims. I think it would be a very smart financial move if my clinic also had a pharmacy, people could choose other companies—but really who would, when you have all that convenience?

I watched two videos on line about the injections, and I am scared. All the medications, including the birth control pills, function to control and direct my hormones into a very specific path so the doctors can predict and create the best possible outcome for us. It is so bizarre. I mean, don't get me wrong, I am extremely grateful to have this opportunity available to me, but this is so nerve wracking.

I asked Tim last night how this was making him feel. I needed to know he was scared and feeling, in his own way, the way I was. He listed off how anxious and nervous he was about all of this, what if it doesn't work, what if it does but we have a miscarriage and are crushed, how many times do we try after our three that are covered by insurance, how will I handle all of this, the money, all of it. I can honestly say I was happy to hear his long list. He is so solid and stable for me, I was concerned that I was doing all the worrying.

You are supposed to run your own race. Don't you do best, though, when you have a teammate?

December 30, 2010

I got an email from our nurse, we counted wrong! I do not have to take a third pack! I started pack two on December 28th, and January 17th is the last day of active pills and the 18th is my ultrasound and blood work to see where we are at for beginning the cycle and also that morning, I have signed us up for our injection class that same day. I was pretty happy at this luck! Yes, luck; I finish my pack of birth control pills the day I get back from a vacation and was able to schedule my first official IVF appointment and injection class for the same day and do not need to take additional time off for it. Yes, celebrate the small victories!

Another victory, this one far greater—our medications for cycle one, so far came in at $95. I know! I actually called back and double checked; these medicines cost six thousand dollars. The pharmacist told me I had excellent insurance. Okay, reason one to keep my head down and just do my job—no more squeaky wheel gets the oil attitude for this Miss Mouth, they are paying for my baby chances.

In my research of pharmacies I learned that it is quite common for them to have what they call the *donation shelf.* Basically for those whose insurance do not cover the outrageous price of fertility meds pharmacies often accept unused medicines from previous patients. I am unaware as to how one qualifies to be a recipient of these medications—but it is there to help. I suggest asking.

A part of me felt guilty about the vacation. I know it is silly. I am truly hoping that my winter break, (working at a university has several perks) then our vacation will prime my body for relaxation and that I may be able to handle the stressors of being an IVF patient. I have not told work about any of this, nor do I feel I need to right now. There is enough stress about this, why invite others to add to it?

January 12, 2011

We are in the middle of our cruise vacation. We have left Baltimore, done some of Florida and we are currently on our way to the Bahamas. I have dubbed this vacation my Mardi Gras, the holiday before Ash Wednesday when Catholics get fat and happy on donuts before the Lenten season. I am enjoying all the food I want, the alcohol and soaking in every bit of rest, sleep, outings and adult pleasures before my *Lenten sacrifice* of infertility treatments. Our next stop: in vitro fertilization.

I do not ignore the fact that I am truly blessed to have this opportunity. The timing worked out for us, the finances—we are even out with another couple we know—I am blessed, I know that, and I wish that for every infertile couple in the world. This is a struggle, you need a respite; a place for your ego, mind and body to just stop and say, ok, this is rough, but I will be okay.

Yesterday I lounged by the pool and read, today we did lots of touristy things, but what captured me most, was the vegetation of Key West, Florida. The trees specifically, their roots were massive and rough, they meant something. They had lived a rough life, they were amazing—they went wherever they needed, they supported massive trunks, flower and some even lighting units and we took their pictures. I pointed out these marvelous works of nature and we all paused to look. They struck me. Their beauty was not where normal tree beauty is—it did not drop in the autumn and get reborn in the spring, it was here the whole time. I have been here the whole time. Beauty is in the roots, the growth.

You have experiences so you can share them.

January 14, 2011

Vacation has been perfect. Each day has had its own wonderful attributes. I have been able to look at our life positively, I have eaten well, worked out and done vast amounts of nothing.

It was a chilly, windy day and the sun did not come out until our husbands gave up and left my friend and me to lounge on the beach. I was looking at the amazing ocean and decided to do my rosary, and had the urge to put my feet in the water. I stood in the crystal clear water up to my knees. I was still and quiet. There were gentle, soft currents of movement and then, without warning, a sting ray swam up to me, caressing my calf and then moved right in front of me. It was about a foot away for a short amount of time. I did not yell, startle or cause any other disturbance—but I wanted everyone to share it with me. That moment, I need to keep with me, remember it when I seek peace, solace and wonder. My stingray moment.

January 24, 2011

It is like we are walking on a street. Tim and I are sometimes hand in hand, sometimes not. The street has no line down the middle of it, and we are headed somewhere, we both know the way. But we have to dodge the cars coming at us, and look over our shoulder to watch out for the cars coming up behind us. I know we are traveling together, but sometimes I feel like I am walking alone. I think that I feel he can leave me in the street at any moment, so I want to hold his hand, and he lets go. He has never left me; I don't know why I feel he will. I guess I feel since it is my body, that I am more invested in this. I wonder if that makes him feel helpless. There is much he is doing for us, finances are his burden and he does his best to make sure I do not worry. He has been extremely calm and caring, I have no reason to believe he will leave me. I am concerned; I never thought I would face infertility, so the unknown is scary to me. I have flashes of doubt. I feel that if I lay the groundwork of doubt it won't hurt so badly if it happens. I am being unfair.

Stop thinking. Love him, simply love him.

January 31, 2011

This is a gift, damn it. I have been given the opportunity to meet myself and know God. I have the chance of moving through this with grace and showing others the beauty of crisis. I am not being punished, sometimes, things just happen to people. It is how you respond and get through them which can define you— not the incident. I have the ability to make infertility known, talked about and maybe even comfort someone. I can speak up for infertility, I will speak up for infertility.

I want to pause here, to reflect that God isn't for everyone. I already shared my husband is an atheist. I cannot tell you how many fertility books I read basically saying the path to fertility was prayer. It was annoying, and to me even foolish. I need science. I need to follow directions. I need prayer for my brain, to talk to someone without judgment about how jealous and ugly I felt, for me, that was God. I have no one to share an ugly vent to. God isn't the path to fertility, but I think for some, faith provides the therapy while science provides the path.

Finish.

My infertility was like running full speed, then taking a face-plant into gravel. I lay there motionless while the others race past me gaining ground, as I stare off knowing that I lost, and the searing pain taking hold. Everything hurts, but I don't yet understand the extent of my injuries. My eyes flutter and I realize I can get up on my own. I flinch, the others running at a full clip, roll over and instead of jumping up and sprinting towards the finish line trusting that the bits and shards of gravel will just fly off, I roll. I curl up into a fetal position, protecting myself from the others and as I hoist myself up to standing I slowly and meticulously brush off the bits and shame. I am vertical. I can be seen, so they rush around me. I start over, but with a different plan.

I am present. I see the roads before me when they present themselves. I see those passing by, and notice them. I feel the weather and hear my breath. I run again. I have no idea what my finish line will look like, but I can only hope for greatness and run my own race, one moment at a time.

No one *understands* what you are going through unless they have run this particular race. Your significant other will react and handle each hurdle differently than you and that is not a fault and should not be treated as such. That being said, it is easier said than done.
I found that no one's reactions were sufficient. There were some who I felt did not react enough and I felt that they simply did not care and I did not want to see them.

But, everyone has a different approach, a different gait, a different mantra—I can't expect perfection from anyone…including me.

First attempt.

The night before my Lupron evaluation we are back from vacation; the dryer was humming, dishwasher running, a doggy snoring and a husband lay in bed reading. I am nervous and scared but full of filthy hope. I say my prayers and do some writing and know that positive thoughts will get me through this with grace.

You are never given more than you can handle.

We will be up early, out the door by six—for there is snow falling currently and this appointment is not to be missed.

It is morning; the roads in our little neighborhood were a sheet of glassy ice. It was freezing rain, and we decided to leave the house at 6:15am for my 7:30 am appointment. We arrived near 7am and soon after I was called in the back room for my blood work first. Tim went with me. He stood in the doorway chewing on his nicotine gum watching the nurse draw a vial of blood. I was calm and I was trying to be positive.

We then move to the back hallway holding space prior to being moved into the examination room. Tim asked if there would be space for him in the next room we would be in, I responded with the affirmative, but to me it felt like he was annoyed.

I ignored what I thought he was feeling, I can't please everyone and I need to be positive at every moment. I chalked it up to him quitting smoking, today, of all days. I need him. I need us to be at our absolute best through this, I need to lean on him, we need to talk to each other and be lovingly honest with each other. But, right now his annoyance vibe makes me want to punch him in the face…lovingly, of course.

We went into the exam room and Tim saw the routine of undressing from the waist down, and hopping up onto the exam bed of butcher paper and how I covered myself with the paper napkin table cloth. He sat down in the chair in the corner.

The doctor and nurse came in for the ultrasound portion. It was more uncomfortable this time, I felt tense and nervous. A cyst was discovered on my ovary. The doctor said that it would need to be drained with a needle, inserted vaginally. (I have never knowingly had a cyst.) I was to go to the front office, get an appointment for today: *a cyst aspiration*. My nurse would call me later this afternoon for my blood work results, if my estrogen was elevated—because of my cyst, we could not start my medication protocol and possibly wait until my next cycle to start our first IVF attempt.

With this threat of another hurdle, I made the appointment for 1:45pm, there was a 10:30am slot open, however, we had a scheduled injection class from 9 to 11am.

The class was with another couple and my nurse with the shaved head and tattoos—I felt comforted by her. We learned about each injection medication, I did a practice shot with saline, and we practiced mixing some of the vials and I asked the questions I had without hesitation. This was not the time to be shy and worry about saying something stupid. We first practiced handling the needles on a used piece of foam rubber, we then practiced bunching up the fat on our belly—this would be our injection sites. I move with confident ease—that confidence when something else takes over, when you actually have nothing left to lose; when you harness your *Tricky* self.

There are many fertility medications; each combination is tailored to fit the patients' needs. The following details my protocol, in conjunction with thyroid medication.

Strangely with infertility, most protocols begin with birth control pills. Yes, in order to conceive you must first go on a pack of birth control pills. I meet this with confusion too, prior to this my knowledge and perception of *the pill* was not one of controlling hormones, but of preventing pregnancy. I think now of how foolish I have been regarding my health; instead of researching, advocating and being my own health expert, I followed what was suggested. Do what everyone else did.

The pills they prescribe are low estrogen, and seem generic, no name, store brand bottom shelf type of estrogen.

The Lupron microdose is a small vial that needs refrigeration. It requires a rather equally small needle normally used for insulin in those with type one diabetes. (Spoiler: you are going to have a favorite gauge needle.) The vial or jar has a rubber top, so this medication is the one that makes me most feel like a drug addict. With this one you learn to flick the needle to rid it of air bubbles. Because I take this one twice a day I get used to it quickly, though with so many injections, my abdomen does start to display my secret with small red dots.

Follistim is administered as though Batman invented it. The drug itself is in a vial, shaped much like the sample perfume bottles adhered obnoxiously into magazines (when magazines existed). It also needs refrigeration. The drug perfume vial is dropped into a pen shaped device. You dial your dosage using a click wheel and at each injection you swap out a small needle. This drug is often overfilled, so it can feel like Chanukah…you think the vial is done, but nope, you have one more dose left before changing the cartridge.

Menopur is chemistry class. It is a powdered tablet in a small jar, and depending on your dosage is how many tablet(s) to saline you mix using a needle, then swapping for a smaller needle before you inject yourself. This one is very labor intensive, and of course the one I need to do in the evenings, while at work… The mixing is done using needles, as if they are suction tools; you pull the saline from one jar, and discharge it into the other one containing the powdered tablet, then swirl it-swap needles, then shoot it.

hCG is the shot in the butt that Tim has to give me. This is lovingly called the *trigger shot*, it triggers the follicles to mature—this is done 35 hours prior to egg retrieval. Typically the clinic will have an estimate date when you will need to trigger and will draw a target on your butt during your monitoring appointment, send you home, and call you with the result confirming what time to administer the shot that night or maybe the next day. The needle is much larger than the others—like a serious drug addict—and once it is done, there are no other shots to do. This is also the shot that is the reason you cannot take a home pregnancy test before your official blood pregnancy test. Home tests are looking for the presence of hCG, which this shot gives you artificially, so to speak. So you must wait a dreaded two weeks after your embryo transfer to find out if you got lucky, and are indeed pregnant.

Endometrin is a tablet you administer vaginally with a stick. Imagine a tampon, but instead of two parts—the plunger and the holder, it is just one piece. You balance (yes, it doesn't quite fit the holder) the large tablet in the holder, and shove it in. It is as gross and awkward as it sounds—and even more icky because it leaks a chalky antacid like discharge. I wear a panty liner; in fact during the majority of the testing and monitoring time I need one, it seemed I was leaking something out of my vagina at all times, I cannot reiterate this enough.

To get pregnant I ate clean, cut out caffeine, cut alcohol, cut recreational drugs, and then promptly became a genius at sneaking self injections in a bathroom stall at work.

The injection class finished at 10:24am and we went back to the main office to ask if that 10:30am cyst aspiration slot was still open. It was, I signed the consent form describing the process, used the restroom and at 10:45am I went into another examination room. Tim stayed in the waiting room. I thought there would be anesthesia as listed on the consent forms.

The doctor and nurse came in and I assumed the position; feet in the stirrups and the Hail Mary running through my head. I felt the speculum opening and I heard him talking to me—but he has a bit of a Spanish accent that I could not decipher over the loud buzz of the fluorescents. I felt the transvaginal ultrasound slide in and there was a lot of pressure. Then he asked if he should go fast or slow, I responded fast—because I had no idea what was to happen next.

The most intense pressure and pain entered my body. I actually let out a *yelp*. My eyes began to water and I cried with pain. It was sharp and as if too many tampons were placed sideways inside my body. He talked to me during the procedure, but honestly, I did not care, I wanted it to be over.

When it was done, I think they said they pulled 20 cc of fluid from the cyst. I am not sure. I had a very hard time sitting up afterwards, I felt extreme cramping and it felt as if there was a foreign object, horizontally, inside me. I was re-assured that there was nothing in there. I cried.

I gathered the courage I had, got dressed and headed into the hall where I was greeted by three nurses whom all comforted me. My case nurse was there too and playfully yelled at my doctor for *hurting her Mary*. He told me that the other way of doing it was more of an operating room procedure and often worst, he then offered his kidney area for me to punch. I told him I would save them up… One of the nurses suggested I kick him in the balls.

We can send a man to the moon, I have a phone that can pinpoint my location within 5 feet and the methods of fertility testing, gynecology and cyst aspiration are this? Seriously? Ahem, this is why we need women in charge of all the things…

I cried some more, on our way home Tim filled my antibiotic prescription, got me Tylenol and surprised me with three bars of dark chocolate. I took my antibiotic, the Tylenol and headed to bed. He made me pork roll and eggs—we figure I should get my fill of nitrates and salty meats before shit gets serious. I love pork roll. He made the most delicious garlicky eggs and a slice of rice bread toast. (NJ alert: it is pork roll, not Taylor ham.)

Tim joined me for a nap, of about two hours. I checked my voicemail around 3:30pm and heard the good news; my estrogen and all other levels were good. We were cleared to start our protocol. I called my nurse back to ask a few questions I had, and she wanted to make sure that I was okay after this morning's procedure. I told her that the Tylenol and a nap helped a bunch.

I entered my medication notes in both my phone and our fridge calendar. Protocol day one of my Lupron micro dose is Thursday, the 20th. And so it begins. I can do this.

When I was listening to the voicemail, I gave Tim the thumbs up. He smiled and began dancing. Not well, mind you, but dancing a happy dance.

I called my mom and told her about today. She told me that after everything I have been through pushing out a baby will be no problem.   She told me she was proud of me and that she would say the rosary for me. We will see them and my little brother this weekend. I am loved. I know this. I can do this. Now, some dinner, chocolate…

January 19, 2011
'Twas the night before injections and I was checking my stock
To see if I had all the things that I needed
But oh, my! Gasp! What a shock!
I have no alcohol wipes, I shout, appalled!
To CVS I go, Bailey angry at me,
"I am sorry ma'am, these are recalled."
But, how can that be?
To Walgreens I go, in search of wipes.
"Recalled, ma'am", and even the lady behind me gripes!
But they are so convenient! And so many injections to come...
So with a bottle of alcohol and lint-free rounds I head on home.
I tell Tim the mess
But we agree, let's not panic, this is only a test.

January 20, 2011
First injections were today, Tim was with me for the morning one, and came home from work as I was doing the evening one. As far as I know, him seeing me do the injections is what is keeping him from smoking—and the nicotine gum is helping too. I want to do whatever I can to help him with it—but I need to take care of myself too!

January 21, 2011
Surprisingly, this mornings' shot was a bit easier—I was also

slightly rushing to work, but I found that taking a calming breath as I stab myself, helped.

I have not told work of my plight. A thought occurred to me that maybe it is none of their business. So far no appointments will interfere with my work and the date of retrieval and transfer are unknown at this time—so I can't prepare them yet, and next week when I am working late and need to do injections at work no one else will be around, so there is a possibility I can get through our first attempt unnoticed...

What stinks is that normal people can try, conceive, and have the luxury of not disclosing information until they are in the clear and healthily pregnant. And, by that time, no employer can fire you for being pregnant; it is a given you will have maternity leave, mood swings and doctor appointments. Whereas infertility is a secret subject that no one talks about. Like I am somehow a freak to be going to the lengths we are going to even to try to conceive. It makes me feel so vulnerable, exposed and yet no one knows.

We have no idea what someone else may be going through in their life. How quickly I used to judge others. It is amazing what you learn about yourself in your darkest hours.

Let me get through today with grace.

January 22, 2011

Today totaled four injections. You have to be a rocket scientist to go through IVF—how fair is that?

Okay, listen up, everyone who is dumb as a bag of hammers, you to this side of the room—you will have the ability to conceive via the Neanderthal method and get to use intercourse. Those of you whom are left will have to undergo a multitude of testing, inappropriate touching and prodding by a plethora of doctors followed by self administered subcutaneous injections in which you will mix the dosing yourself without a medical degree…

Awesome. Maybe I got in the wrong line….

I have two injections, then church and two more tonight after dinner.

I am a bad ass. I am *Tricky Cervix*. I have had a cyst aspiration with no anesthesia and I am currently administering costly drugs to myself via injections! It takes one hell of a chick to do this! God bless the women of IVF—or any battle with infertility for that matter! We kick ass! Sometimes you need to be your own cheerleader.

Tim reminded me that within two weeks will be our transfer appointment—retrieval too. Crazy. This is a huge responsibility, not only the giving over of my body to give life, but the commitment to go through this medical process with grace and faith. The responsibility lies within maintaining a positive outlook, remaining kind to others, giving thanks and expressing true patience.

January 24, 2011

This morning was Lupron microdose and my third Follistim injection (Batman device). According to the math, I should have had to put in a new cartridge today—my dosage is 225 and there is 600 per cartridge. Well, I got the full dose today! I thought the pen messed up, or was broken. I wanted to mess with it and see if I dialed another number if more would come out or if I could troubleshoot the pen. But I decided to ask the nurses at my appointment if there is more medication then listed in the cartridge.

It was like Chanukah!

I had my 7:30am blood work only appointment, and sure enough, the cartridges are over filled and on my next dose, I will finish that one, change out the cartridge and finish the dose.

I will get a call this afternoon telling me what today's results say and what my evening dosage will be as well as when my next appointment will be. Basically, from this point on, I know nothing and will be told exactly what to do day to day. (This is specifically when you need your Type A and Type B pants on.) It is a bit nerve wracking—especially because I still have a full time job. It would be lovely to take a year sabbatical; go through this, get pregnant, deliver then decide if I want to go back or not... but that will not happen. *You never know what someone is going through...*

It is amazing that I have been taking this all one day at a time, and it actually feels like it is flying by. I guess that is also how mothers feel watching their children grow up so fast, it always felt that disappointments lingered while joy raced by, but I guess, it is all in your perspective. You can embrace any moment you chose.

I am told my estrogen seems to be higher than it should be at this time. Currently it is 82, they want me back tomorrow for an ultrasound and blood work—they want to see if they are moving too fast with me.

I have no clue what they are talking about. I trust that they do, I have to.

January 25, 2011

Lupron and Follistim in the morning, then blood work and an ultrasound. I felt like an expert waiting in the waiting room. It was busy this morning, lots of other women waiting for their own monitoring appointment. I saw them all as potential friends. Many seemed close to my age, I feel for them. This morning, Tim, was the only guy there. Often there is another male partner in the waiting room, occasionally he will let out a sigh and has a look of mixed boredom and apathy. Not a fair description, I know. If they are in that room they are truly supportive, and want a child just as much as their female partner. The male species just seems to respond to many things differently. Maybe they feel helpless and in that feeling, they express it as boredom. The presence of smart phones have caused this boredom to appear even more bored and apathetic, as if whatever is on the phone is exponentially more interesting than trying to conceive. It is part offensive, and part expected. I too am guilty of checking my phone while waiting for my name to be called. Stewing over dread is detrimental, checking in on social media to see what everyone else is eating, may be a bit healthier.

They do the ultrasound first, I have no cysts, and the doctor counts out a total of five follicles. I sense the dismay, and I know five is not the number they were looking for. For those playing the home version of this game; a normal woman puts out ten to twelve follicles each month—and currently I am on medication to put out more…so where the fuck are they? Apparently they were expecting sixteen to twenty follicles from me.

At that moment, I simply think to myself, well, at least I have five. Being positive sometimes requires a shoulder shrug and an *at least…*

I go in for my blood work and the nurses are kind. She comments on the bruise on my left arm, I explain that I named that one, *Labcorp*.

Traffic is bad when we leave and by the time we get home I rush to help pack Tim a lunch and get his coffee together while he cleans up and leaves for work. I am working evenings this week, so that is one burden off my plate—well, except that I am really tired and since I don't work normal people hours, I have to do the night time injections at work along with not sleeping in because of the morning blood monitoring appointments…but I digress…

I get antsy around 3:30pm and decide to take my phone for a walk. I walk around the building at work and realize the magnitude of shit I am going through and that no one (only one person) at work knows it. The drama that goes on is insane! I have learned through this, how asinine people can be. Really, we need to have another meeting about where the audience chairs are going to be placed?

While pacing the building, my phone picks up more bars and tells me I have a voicemail from 2pm. It is the nurse covering for my case nurse telling me that *I have five follicles, my estrogen was at 166 and to keep the dosages the same but return in two days for another ultrasound and blood work.*

I call her, make sure I understand my medication doses and schedule my next appointment. She seems nice.

It is time for my evening injections, and more people are in my work office than expected. I thought I would be alone in the evenings; I could store my Lupron in the fridge with no issues. Not a chance.

I stealthily get my meds out of the fridge like a ninja, I keep it in a resalable container, my prescriptions are wrapped in paper towels in the container so it looks like I packed lunch or dinner. I pull my other meds from my purse, and put some alcohol wipes in my pockets. (My mom found wipes at home in NJ, turns out only some were re-called! She is a great mom!) I leave my sharps container in my purse, too big for the trip to the dressing room. (I am not a take my purse to the bathroom kind of woman, so it would be more suspicious if I suddenly take my purse with me, it would appear like I was leaving to go home, which I was not.) I am doing this all out in the open. About a year ago, a boss decided that our office needed to be *more inviting*, so they took all our cubicle walls. There is one dividing me and a co-worker but I face the door, so I positioned my chair and did all this without her seeing outright. Then again, she is diabetic, so she may have recognized my sleek pencil case holding syringes and medicines…she said nothing. I head for a dressing room on the other side of the building and simply (filthy) hope no one comes in. I figure, whoever unlocks the door, actually works for me, and I am fairly certain I can say, *I take self injected medicine, no one knows, please keep this matter private*, and that would be okay. It is clearly not heroine I am taking…I mean I don't have a spoon or anything…

I am getting better at the menopur, but man, it is a pain to mix it. (Menopur is the powder tablet that is mixed with saline via a syringe.) The Lupron (feel like an addict) is a piece of cake now.

I get home that night and I am so very tired. I head upstairs and Tim asks what he can do for me, I request ice cream and peanut butter. He brings it up to me, we talk about our days and I eat. I request a second bowl. We talk some more and he tells me that I look tired and should go to bed; we have to take my car to the shop in the morning and I need to do my shots, so I still need to get some rest. I watch some TV and lay with Bailey, our dog. I neglect to turn off the lights, brush my teeth or take out my contacts.

About an hour later, according to Tim; he comes up, sees the light on and heads to the bathroom. He sees that my contact lens case is open and empty. He comes in the room, sees Bailey kick me and my head lifts. Apparently, he tried to convince me to fully go to bed and not simply lay on top of the covers with my contacts in and the lights on. It was at that moment that I decided to no longer keep my head up and it falls back to the pillow. He coaxes me to get ready for bed, I do and fall fast asleep.

These hormones are making me sleepy.

January 26, 2011

I woke up this morning to surprise snow accumulation. I was scheduled to be at work around 4pm, but the university closed for the day at 3pm. So I had an unintentional day off—even though I spent most of it on the phone or dealing with email to figure out a contingency plan; we were supposed to have a technical rehearsal for a dance piece.

Today is my parent's anniversary. I called them and they sounded good. They too are in the midst of this snow storm. My mom asked how things were going and I told her where we were at. I know she does not want me to have to go through this, what mother would? She asked if because I was high on estrogen could something happen on its own.

My mom is a registered nurse. She currently works in hospice and used to be a labor and delivery nurse. And, she had ten children of her own. We are both learning about IVF through this, and many talk about how things *happen on their own,* or that they *know someone who after they tried for so long, they adopted, then they got pregnant on their own.* Those stories are wonderful, and I have hope, and I don't know everything. But, sometimes those stories and hopes are hurtful. They make me feel like the speaker thinks I am making the wrong decision. Honestly, there are times that no one can say anything right to me. This is such a delicate balance for those around me and for me too.

January 27, 2011

We lost power while I was asleep; Tim came in and put an extra blanket on me and the bed. Losing power also means losing heat. We woke up to no power and to about 8 or 9 inches of snow on the ground.

I opened the fridge to do my shots, and it hits me that my meds need to be stored under 46 degrees! I quickly pull them, do my shots by candle light at 6am in the morning and we agree later that we will stick the meds and some food items in a cooler outside—I stash the thermometer in there too.

Tim shovels the end part of our driveway were the plow-wall is while I clean off the car. (I clean off the entire car, roof included. Seriously people, clean off the roof of your car! Your roof snow flies off and hits the cars behind you, making you an utter jerk.) Did I mention the car I am cleaning off is the one that does not have a defroster, nor heat? Yeah, that car is the one we have to take to the fertility clinic today. The good car, my car, is currently at the mechanics getting a lot of expensive things done and it was not ready yesterday afternoon before the snow started.

We drive to the clinic and on our way we lose count at 30 cars abandoned on the side of the road that has since been plowed in. The storm was terrible last night, I feel sorry for those people. A tow truck works to remove them, one by one.

I think to myself about the premise that if you go to a fertility doctor or you seek fertility treatments you have given up. People say that using IVF or any fertility treatment is playing God. I think about this and know that it is simply not true. How can one possibly say that I have given up? At this point I have given myself twenty-eight subcutaneous injections, been on thyroid medication for five months, had more blood draws than I can count, more transvaginal ultrasounds and other devices shoved into my vagina like a porn star all while still holding a full time job, being a nice person, keeping my sense of humor and being a great wife—after years of trying naturally with ovulation kits, thermometers and examining my egg white cervical mucus—all because I want to have a baby. I want the opportunity to attempt to have a baby. I want to exhaust all possibilities to have a baby, a child, to be the best damn mother I can be. How is this giving up? How is this taking the easy route? And how, can I possibly do all this without my faith, my faithfulness and trust that God is holding me up in all of this, that She is guiding my doctors and my path. How could I do this without my filthy hope and faith? And if I did not believe in God and still went through all of this, what does it matter to anyone how I go about trying to conceive? It is none of their damn business.

I have met myself in these dark moments.

January 28, 2011

I hear a metronome ticking. The precise tick tock of the clock keeping us all on beat.

The routine morning shots at home then an ultrasound and blood work appointment. It seemed to go well, and I pause to notice the busy pace of the morning monitoring routine; it is amazing the different women dealing with the same issue. From all walks of life women streamed in, headed to the counter, filled out the sign in and information sheet, greeted the receptionists and took a seat. We know the routine, we all sit in the waiting room during monitoring hours—listening to the tick tock…we are all there to go into an exam room, undress from the waist down, get probed, get dressed and wait in the hall for blood to be drawn. Tick tock.

In my heart, I am friends with every one of them. We have all experienced the devastation of learning we cannot get pregnant naturally, no matter what the medical reason is, here we are, all engaged in the same morning monitoring routine. Tick tock. *The counter, sign in, second sign in, greet the receptionist, take a seat, hear your name, follow the staff into an exam room, undress from the waist down, wait, get probed, get dressed, wait in the hall for blood to be drawn.* Tick tock.

Anyone who marvels at the efficiency of Chick Fil A drive thru has never been a fertility patient—morning monitoring nurses and protocols, now that shit is efficient.

The snow is lightly falling now, and I will be headed to work for a long night, tomorrow is a two-show day, then I am off for two days. I am looking forward to it.

I ordered more Menopur this morning, I have only four doses left, and my doctor is not sure if I will need more or not; being that it is Friday, I would rather order now, than be anxious about it on Monday. The pharmacy was very kind and easy to work with—I ask several questions, and I request more of the Lupron microdose needles.

My abdomen is sore today, and I am noticing that my instinct is not to lift any heavy things or move too fast—this is not normal for me. Not too long ago I was running 20-25 miles in a week, now I am not running at all, but I have done some walking as my nurse suggested. I have to wear my roomier jeans; I am swollen, bloated, and tender. I know I am bigger and I am extremely emotional. There was a story on the news about the Challenger disaster that took place twenty-five years ago today; I began to weep in the car. Tim, held my hand and smiled at me.

I told him, "These hormones are killin' me!" I think I cry once a day.

I am debating telling my co-workers what I am going through. I am to the point that I believe they deserve to know, but only if the opportunity to tell them presents itself. I need to be positive,

calm and focused. It is amazing; I know that in a year, this will
be just another difficult moment in my life that I have gone
through, another thing that has added to my character. For now, I
need to take it all one day at a time. We are one day closer.

Report: my estrogen is at 667 and all five follicles are maturing
nicely! I am to keep the same dosage and see them on Sunday—
but at another location. Turns out the clinic (which is located in a
hospital) has a water main problem and they are fixing it this
weekend, so all monitoring is going to their other locations. To
Annapolis we go.

January 29, 2011

*Shots this morning, then I went back to bed. I have a two show
day today and needed some sleep. I am feeling quite strange. I
wouldn't call it bloating, but there is a definite tenderness and
largeness to my abdomen. I am finding myself a bit slower and
hesitant to do much bending and lifting—in fact none at all. I
think it is time to tell my coworkers, we are getting close to "shot
in the butt day" and I do not foresee my days off lining up with
when my retrieval and implant days… maybe…time to come out
to them.*

I missed my opportunity to tell them…oh well…

January 30, 2011

I did shots this morning, then to an appointment in Annapolis—
quite a lovely experience. We are fortunate that the group we
chose is well organized, clean and has high success rates.

Around 4pm I got the call. My estrogen is at 978, we are to
trigger tonight at 10pm, I am no longer to take the Lupron
microdose, menopur or follistim—I am done with them. We
trigger tonight, have a *post trigger* appointment at 7:30 am
tomorrow morning then on Tuesday at 10am is retrieval! Holy
schmoly—we were not expecting this to be today! I thought they
would draw the target on my butt (so Tim can inject in the correct
spot) when we were getting close, but apparently, you got to be
ready for anything.

Tim seems nervous, I am too, but we have come so far. I counted
it up; I have done 40 injections, who knows how many
appointments. I believe I have done all I can. It is fitting that I
now must leave it in the hands of Tim, his sperm, my doctors and
nurses and trust that God will guide them.

Well, it hurt like it would when a doctor would give me a shot in
the upper butt—so I guess he did it right. I lay on the bed with no
bottoms on; he asked me if I was ready. I felt the cold alcohol
wipe on my skin, then I felt the stab. He talked me through what
he was doing, how he was pulling up on the plunger to check if
he hit a vein, he did not, then, he pushed the medication in, and
told me he was done. I felt him exhale.

I got up to put my pajama pants on, and lay back on the bed, he
lay beside me and said I love you.

"We just played doctor!" I said

We laughed. I crawled under the covers with my book and he
brought me a glass of water.

January 31, 2011

*We have a morning appointment, and there are no shots for me to
take! I was afraid, that out of habit I would inject myself so last
night I packed up my meds and asked Tim to leave me a note next
to the coffee pot reminding me to not do any shots.*

*I walked into the kitchen this morning, and on the coffee pot there
was a note: SHOTS: NO! COFFEE: YES!*

We do the normal blood work and ultrasound—but every nurse
and doctor greets us a bit warmer and tells us *good luck*. I think I
even heard music in the background, possibly cartoon birds
singing. Tomorrow is a big day.

All five of my follicles are looking good. We will hear this
afternoon the status of my levels.

After the ultrasound we meet with another nurse and she goes over the protocols for the next few days. Tonight is an antibiotic and nothing to eat or drink after midnight, like a Mogwai. She suggests lots of fluids today to make the IV and tomorrow's procedure a bit easier. Tim's contribution, takes place in the morning, followed by my part. There is a lot of information to go over, she explains it very well to us, but it is overwhelming.

We leave with future appointments on the books, several *good lucks* and a semen collection kit. (This is just a sealed sanitized cup, though a semen collection kit with the cup, porn and a sports drink is not a terrible idea.)

I think if I let the magnitude of what we need to do actually sink in, it will be more stressful. I feel it is my duty to embrace this; to seize this moment and do everything I absolutely can, and accept whatever it is. No, I don't want to have to do this again, but I will. I love my follicles.

When we were little, when we asked of our mom, *where was I before I was born*, she responded, *God's pocket.* I am trusting that She reaches into Her pocket and allows me the privilege to be someone's mommy.

This is just like training, or the night before a long run. I am resting up, drinking a lot of fluids, following the plan and getting support. I will go to bed early, wake up and feel refreshed. I cannot predict the future, I can hope for the best but all in all, it is one foot in front of the other. I will deal with the hurdles when they show themselves. The mantra is, and always should be, to run your own race. We are one day closer.

February 1, 2011

Tim gets to do his part! The roads are not too bad with ice, so we leave around normal time. He fills out the paper and accidently checks the IUI box after first correctly checking the IVF box but second guessing himself. His form looks like a grade school student's mess and he writes in; *I really mean this one*, next to IVF with an arrow. We laugh. There is a moment that I think to myself, after all this—you don't remember what fertility treatment we are going through? I decide not to not start that battle.

We pull up to the clinic and joke about his form. Then I ask if he has his sample. It is in his coat pocket, but we joke as if we left it at home on the kitchen counter.

"Can I have another cup and a private room? Or, at the very minimum, a cup?"

I actually double over and laugh out loud at this in the parking lot. It feels good. It was the cathartic release I needed.

I am called to the pre-op room. I have been told to not wear any jewelry, contacts or scented bath products. I feel naked without my wedding ring, but cute in my glasses. A nurse asks me to change into two hospital gowns, one to wear with open part to the back, the other like a robe. Again, with the hospital gowns, the missing snaps, super knotted ties and the extra-extra large size, my nemesis! I dramatically wave my arms in disdain at the hospital gowns before getting undressed. Once I figure it out, I slip on the hair net and brown socks. I sit. I think positive thoughts about my follicles. I imagine them being healthy, squishy and perfect.

A nurse comes in and asks me many, many questions. It is as if they have zero medical history on me, which drops in a seed of doubt to my mind. She starts an IV on me, I think it is supposed to make me calm, and it does. (I would like a refill to take home.) I no longer doubt the line of questioning I endured. Later my anesthetist comes in the room; she has an Irish accent and a name I can't remember. She asks me more questions. They both ask me my weight and height, and I can't help but wonder why getting on a scale is not part of this assessment. I could totally lie about my weight and screw up the medicine she gives me. Which, in this case, lying about your height and weight would be tragic. She tells me she will be administering Propofol, which is the same drug that killed Michael Jackson. This does not comfort me. She does not tell me the Michael Jackson connection, it just jumps into my head on its own.

I pray a Hail Mary for every nurse and doctor I met. I needed them to do their absolute best. I am moved into the operating room, with a second potty trip on the way. They need you to have an empty bladder. I lay down, monitors are put on me and that is the last thing I remember…

I wake up in the recovery room and asked how I am feeling and if I have any pain. I have cramping, but it is not bad, I tell her a 3 or a 4 on the pain scale. She later gives me extra-strength Tylenol and cranberry juice. I had three cups there. I could not leave until I had urinated. I felt tired and chatty but had no problems peeing, and no blood in the toilet. I had very little spotting, but that was okay according to them. Tim came back to see me, then I got dressed and a ride in a wheelchair as Tim pulled the car around front to take me home.

We got home, I got right into pajamas and under the covers. Tim came up with water for me. I fell asleep while he was making me breakfast, but I woke up when he came in the room. I ate, and then fell back asleep for four hours. I woke up for dinner and some chat time with Tim and later my mom on the phone, then back to sleep.

February 2, 2011

This afternoon I got a message! Yesterday, they aspirated five follicles, and got five mature eggs! All five eggs had ICSI performed on them and today we have three of which are embryos!

I am hopeful, and yet depressed. This low number, I know is not the norm. But, we only need one right? I love those embryos. I want to be a good home for them, I want to be able to do this.

I had to explain to my boss that I would need additional time off, but did not tell him what the procedure was. He did not ask if I was okay, he merely scoffed when I said I was not sure exactly what day the medical procedure would be scheduled. (In case it was not clear, we do not have a great working relationship.)

Frankly, it is none of his business. If I say I may need these dates off for medical reasons—and I have an enormous bank of leave, then really, there should not be a problem. Yes, I am defensive. One day maybe I will explain, or maybe not.

I finally tell my two close co-workers the truth. They both listened and wished us luck. I don't know why I was so nervous telling them, they have never done anything to intentionally hurt me—I know that we all care a great deal about each other. In all honesty, they are like siblings to me; I should have known they would be supportive. I was just afraid to admit this intimate admission of struggle.

I came home from work overwhelmed and a bit depressed. I had chips, salsa, cheese and ice cream for dinner. Not typical at all for me. This is big. This is an overwhelming ordeal to go through. Tim thought I needed a proper dinner, so he made me eggs and bacon. I make it sound like breakfast is the only meal he can cook…it is…that is all he can cook.

I hear tomorrow about the status of our three embryos and how they did overnight. We will also be told when to report back at the hospital for transfer. Day three will be Friday, and I have already put in for Saturday off as well. I am choosing to stay in bed an extra day. This is tough.

February 3, 2011

Three embryos are still dividing! The nurse called this morning to say they have 4 cells and we should report tomorrow at 9am for our transfer. She gave me medicine orders and told me that there is a chance that tomorrow morning they decide to wait until day 5, which would be a transfer on Sunday. I am rooting for tomorrow, just because, but honestly, I want whatever is best. I have waited this long, I can wait some more. All along I have said the mantra, *we are one day closer*. Here we are, actually one day closer.

I am nervous. I am scared that my embryos will hate my uterus
and not implant. I fear that they will fall out when I get up to pee.
That it will be too hard and I will find myself in a heap of tears
wishing I was single and lonely.

I know the truth. I know that I am a happily married woman
capable of great things. I know that I have come through many
obstacles in life and I know I can do this and whatever else comes
next. I know that something else will come next, I know that life
is full of hurdles and it is my responsibility to leap over them
gracefully…even when it feels like I am a drunk raccoon jumping
from trash can to trash can. Practice.

I have no idea what tomorrow will bring, but I know I will move
through it the best that I can at that time.

February 4, 2011

Transfer day!

*We went to the hospital as planned and sure enough, all systems
were go for transfer! Our two little embryos were at 8 cells and
they will be freezing our third if it continues to do well.*

I sat in the waiting room sipping my water; they need my bladder
to be moderately full for the transfer. Around 9:30 am they
brought me back to a room, I changed into the gowns, (eye roll)
hair cap, socks and waited patiently. Tim was brought back to
wait with me. He had put my purse in the car and came back with
my jacket and water. First the doctor came back. I was told the
status of my embryos. Five follicles were retrieved, five eggs
were found, all five had ICSI performed on them. One fertilized
abnormally, one did not fertilize and three were fertilized and
were doing well. Two would be transferred to me this morning
and they had eight cells, the other one if it goes to *blast* (a
blastocyst is an embryo of 5 to 7 days after fertilization and its
cells are dividing and doing awesome) it will be frozen. I sign off
on the transfer, as does Tim. We wait.

A male nurse comes back to tell me they are ready for me, he asks
how my bladder is, I tell him I need to pee. He is ridiculously

happy about this. He tells Tim and me that he has adopted children and now has a grandchild, he is a happy gentleman who proceeds to talk quite a bit about children. This surprises me, as so far in this experience there has been very little discussion about if any of our medical team are parents or really, any talk about kids at all.

I am brought into a room that looks much like an examination room. There is a stretcher, monitor screen and lots of medical hardware. There is a front and back door to the room; I notice when we came in it was labeled, *IVF Lab*. I am instructed to lay down with my bottom very close to the folded down part of the *bed* and my knees bent onto the stretcher. Basically, in the usual position sans stirrups. He begins to pull my gowns up and explains that they do an on the belly ultrasound for this. I was a bit taken aback. I am used to male doctors waiting to do anything until the female nurse came in. But, I never felt threatened, plus there were people in and out of the room.

The doctor came in. I had the warm, blue ultrasound goo on my belly and was watching on the monitor my very full bladder on what appeared to be old black and white television showing clips of outer space. A nurse came in, asked me to state my name and what was about to happen, basically what I said had to match up with her paperwork. From the corner of my eye I could tell the back door of the exam room led directly into a laboratory.

First came the speculum. I swear, that it is so painful that I wonder if I have an extra flap down there. I wanted to say—*just let me do it!* Next was a catheter (from what I could tell) on the monitor I saw my large, full bladder—which they all complimented me on—and then I did see a thin white line appear. It is hard to understand what I was looking at and I needed to trust that the medical staff knew. Once he was set, he told another nurse to go get the embryos. A moment later he had them. On the monitor I saw what looked like shooting stars move across a tiny space then gather into a circle of white. He then passed what I guess to be a syringe-like device back to the other nurse. The doctor explained that the lab was going to check the device to make sure it is empty; sometimes embryos get stuck. I did not move, and was hoping that during this waiting time they would not try to make small talk with me about my vagina.

The male nurse joked with me,

"I bet you never thought conception would be this uncomfortable!"

I replied, "I never thought conception would be this public, with my husband out in the hallway."

There was laughter throughout the procedure, everyone wanted to make this a happy experience.

The nurse returned and exclaimed, "All clear."

The catheter and speculum slid out, and my belly goo wiped. There were *thank you* and *good lucks* exchanged. Another nurse came to take over for the male nurse, and was surprised that we were done already. The whole thing may have taken ten minutes.

I was rolled back to where I left Tim, this time I was on a stretcher. The nurse told him that at 10:24am I would be able to get up and use the bathroom. She showed him how to release the side rails. She told me that she had done two rounds of IUI. I did not ask about the outcome. She was a sunny lady and wished us luck. Then she left us with instructions I truly appreciated:

"It is out of your hands now, rest here for the full fifteen minutes, and then you can use the bathroom. Don't worry, your cervix is closed up, they will not fall out, no matter the bumps you hit on the ride home. It is out of your hands now. Go home and stay in bed. (To Tim) Feed her well, cause as of right now, (To me) you are pregnant, so Tylenol is okay, but until your test, you are pregnant."

Until your test, you are pregnant.

She walked away, I looked at Tim and I saw what I believe to be my own expression mirrored in his. I saw the reality of that news hit him, the joy, the worry and the gratitude. My eyes started to tear and he held my hand. He held my hand for most of the fifteen minutes.

At 10:26am I had the most frightening trip to the bathroom of my life. Since my bladder was full, it also was the longest, most nervous pee I have ever had. The nurse had reassured me they would not fall out, but gravity works, it is a law. How are my embryos going to stay in there? Does my womb defy gravity, I realize my soon to be released pee is not actually in my uterus, but shouldn't I be horizontal for at least a month?

After I courageously urinated I got dressed and we were released from the hospital. I was able to walk out on my own, which felt weird. It was unreal. I felt like I should be shrouded in caution tape or encased in a life sized bubble at least.

I texted my boss that I would use my personal leave today and tomorrow. I wanted to wait until the procedure was over before I told him I would be out, that way, just in case, I did not need to do any further explaining. (I never did tell him we had IVF.)

Forced bed rest feels very odd. Tim has been the doting husband bringing me food, tea and things to keep me occupied. I know he is nervous, but we must wait. For two weeks; this begins the dreaded *two week wait* when you leave the hospital pregnant, but must wait for a blood test to confirm implantation. And with my IVF protocol I cannot take a home pregnancy test; it will give a positive no matter what because of the trigger shot medication.

I told my parents and my sisters, he told his parents. It is difficult, you want to tell people, but you know full well the gravity of the situation and that it could very likely go the other way. In two weeks we could not be pregnant too.

I still believe this is a gift. How wonderful is it that I am able to do this procedure. That people had the idea, intelligence and the will to discover IVF and create multiple processes that work. That everyone we have come in contact with is all after the same goal; help us conceive and provide all the resources to make sure we are healthy and dealing with this stress. I believe God is involved with this process, I cannot do this without Her, and I know She works through people and science.

How lucky am I to begin these new lives with a proper diet, I know, until told otherwise, that I am pregnant. I know that my health is no longer my own, that I have a responsibility to manage my diet, exercise and stress. All thoughts need to be positive, I have no room for negative junk, I am growing some babies here!

I am fortunate to have this experience. I have had my moments, and I know there will be more, but I also know I will do the very best that I know how in each of those moments. Now, I rest some more. And, we wait.

February 5, 2011

Bloom where you are planted: an appropriate cliché.

I got up and moved around at lunchtime. My butt was pretty sore and I am not used to being in bed for that long. I started to feel stressed, little things were pissing me off. For a brief moment, I thought, oh no, this is period irritation…please don't let it be…

Later in the evening Tim asked if I had done any yoga. I hadn't, I was afraid that I would make some weird movement and kill the embryos. I told him that I would start walking come Wednesday. We are allowed to have intercourse on Wednesday, I figure if I can have sex I should be able to walk on the treadmill—though my discharge papers forbid running or anything high impact. It did say yoga and walking were okay and technically I was only on bed rest yesterday, I gave myself extra bed rest time.

One of my podcasts had a pre-natal yoga class. I figured that was my safest bet. It did relax me and it felt good to move into Warrior II, my favorite pose (not really, I'd rather be in Savasana at any moment in my life) I felt strong. There was one moment in the class where the teacher wanted me to think about my *perfect* body, and how it was *perfectly* formed to carry a child and be a mother. I felt a twinge of anger toward her. Clearly, she did not have the ladies of fertility treatments on her mind…

I ignored my offense and instead moved toward happy thoughts, I even made myself smile and breath a bit deeper.

It is interesting to think about…I went through the training for a marathon for the sheer will to do it, and here I am now, at the mercy of medicines, tests, appointments, hope and sheer emotional determination to get a child. All, within months…

I am at 35 hours after transfer. Implantation takes place between hours 48 and 96. I go back to work in the morning, the goal is to keep my uterus house as welcoming as possible, I imagine my embryos burying themselves into my cozy lining thinking, *I could crash here for a while*. I wonder how strong the power of suggesting positive imagery really is.

February 6, 2011

Back to work, I had to do some light lifting and was so nervous. With this job, things could get interesting for me. I didn't feel comfortable telling anyone in management, and human resources didn't come across as a welcoming bunch.

Being stressed at work is a very common theme for me. I need to work on that.

The great thing about being off caffeine and alcohol is that I sleep wonderfully. Also, I am eating darn well, so my poops are great too. Maybe, I can do this after all.

February 7, 2011

Well, we are in that crucial 48 to 96 hour phase, and I am a bit nervous, but know, it is out of my hands.

I thought about my little shooting stars. I want to use that in their room when decorating. Who cares that it really doesn't go with the Orange Blast that is on the walls…it is special to me.

I did some wonderful yoga tonight and prayer, a whole rosary with the one (I think) my mom gave me for confirmation. It has since broken and five Hail Mary and a Our Father bead is missing, but I adjusted. It felt so light in my hands compared to the other one I have been using. It was almost refreshing.

February 8, 2011

I am feeling really achy and cramped. Last night I used a heating pad and this morning Tim questioned if that is okay. So I emailed my case nurse thinking, of course, it has to be okay—it seems more important to me that he quits smoking! (Yeah, still working on quitting…) However, then online I read several different sites with different opinions on the matter. So now I am confused and worried.

Logically though, few women even know they are pregnant at this phase—they do all sorts of stupid stuff to themselves before they learn they are pregnant. Then again, they did not spend so long trying… I would absolutely hate to learn I harmed the babies because I had a backache.

Last night in my dreams my front tooth fell out. Ask most anyone and they will tell you dreams about teeth falling out are your subconscious telling you a big change in your life is coming. I have had these dreams before, when we moved or I got a new job. I am full of hope, and fear that my heating pad killed my chances…but I had the dream after the heating pad, and I didn't have it on for long…oh jeez, I need to stop thinking!

My nurse emailed me back, sure enough, Tim was right! No heating pads. I have to look over my paperwork and see what else I missed. She encouraged me not to feel bad, it is a common mistake.

While pulling into the parking garage of work I got the voicemail from the clinic. Our third little embryo degenerated and did not make it; it was discarded. I wept. I called Tim, he calmed me down and after we hung up I got a text from him, he loves me.

I went into work, and about my business. In the bathroom stall I prayed for the embryos that did not make it, and I also prayed for the ones that made the cut—I prayed that they could thrive. I feel like they are my last hope, because for now, they are.

February 9, 2011

Day off! I am feeling quite bloated, cramped and tired. I am told it is because my ovaries are working themselves back to their normal size. Today Tim and I are able to have sex, not sure how I feel about that, see above. But it tells me we are in a better place than where we were. Also, in one week is our official pregnancy test. One day closer.

Tim picked up three books, *What to Expect When You Are Expecting*, as well as the same class of book talking about a pregnancy diet and for the daddy to be. Three books he so thoughtfully purchased for us.

I still think it is pretty cool that I know the day we were fertilized. Fighting for this baby, I think, has made me a whole new woman. I fear that this cycle will fail, and I dread doing this again, but I find my positive attitude is more easily accessible these days. I know I could easily talk myself into a rotten mood and wail in a heap of tears, with snot dripping, but I know that tomorrow will be easier.

February 10, 2011

Am I pregnant? It is all I can think about. I know I need to be calm, relaxed and happy. Judgments and anger creep in uninvited into my head and I have fictitious conversations—none of which have happened. I realize I am doing it, close my eyes, begin to breathe deeply and re-start. I need something to keep my mind off of this two-week-waiting period, the cramps, the hope, all of it. How should I prepare myself mentally for the worse? How should I prepare myself for the best?

No matter what I am going through, the sun rises, the wave crash and wind blows. The plants and many animals and bugs are quietly resting right now, but essentially that is what they are made to do. How come humans don't hibernate? I am not sure we are built for this stress, evolution killed us. At least it killed our rest. I need something to re-charge me, engage my passion while I wait. I am sleeping well, I am taking care of myself, I am reading and I am writing. I practice kind self talk. *Do what makes you happy today. You are going through a crisis; ask for help, listen to your body and be happy you are not alone. You have Tim. You have your family and friends. You are one day closer.*

I repeat these positive thoughts all day.

February 11, 2011

Today is my eldest brother's birthday.

I realize the power of suggestion. Here I am thinking that there is a strong possibility that I am pregnant, and just tonight a stereotypical pregnant lady event happened. Tim made macaroni and cheese, a grown up version, gluten free-of course. He put blue cheese in it too. It came out of the oven and I said,

"Whoa, what is that awful smell?"

"Blue cheese?"

"I certainly hope not!"

We ate the meal, it was not great and afterwards I was belching blue cheese. When I went to bed I asked Tim to get me a trash can because I thought I was going to vomit. I also made him wash his hands. I smelled cigarettes and, that too, made me nauseous. He told me it was in my head, because he did not just have a cigarette. It was most definitely not in my head, something smelled bad. (So, this is what happens when Tim cooks something other than breakfast—nausea.)

February 12, 2011

Anger just shows up. Uninvited. Dealing with *her* is taking every ounce of energy I have and frankly I am not interested in wasting all my precious time on these issues. I want happiness. I want joy, the awe and the wonder of life. I want to shout at my anger to *go away*, but I don't know how to do that.

I vacuumed today, I hope that is considered moderate activity and therefore okay for a woman in my *condition*. I am still making a conscious effort to remain calm; in fact I did a little bit of cleaning and then sat on the couch writing for most of the day. I did get dinner started but, by my standards this was a sedentary day.

My mom calls almost every day and some of my sisters are visiting me tomorrow with their kids. My mom claims she is learning a lot about IVF and has even begun reading blogs.

She told me I was currently in the "2ww and it's the pits!"

That is *two week wait*. Yes, it is the pits. I feel stressed and worried and at the same time hopeful and this intense desire to take care of myself. I have not done any blog reading, I was afraid I would be sucked into wallowing instead of moving forward. I tend to find something to sulk about and stay there for too long.

My body feels wrong to me. I am bloated, vaginal suppository medicine is always leaking, I am tired, my belly feels tight and stressed, I have no idea what is going on in there, but I hope magic is happening. This is the down and dirty, filthy, grimy, elbow deep hope I grasp. I hope that nothing I have done in the last eight days has caused the embryos to die. I hope nothing I do in the next four days causes them to die. I hope I can provide a wonderful, hospitable home for them and that they latch on and grow.

February 13, 2011

Today two of my sisters came over with their kids. There were five in the house ranging from 12 to 1. They were noisy, nosy, and messy. I don't know why I vacuumed before they arrived, there are crumbs everywhere, I have to re-launder the tablecloth and the refrigerator magnets are all out of place. Is this what I have been fighting for all this time?

Yes.

I love them all, and was sad that they had to go. As much as it hurts to see people with kids or that their kids are pretty much the sole subjects of conversation. It was fun, they all are so different and I can't wait to meet the little personalities Tim and I made.

I was feeling pretty cramped while they were here, and luckily Tim was Mr. Hospitality. He did all the cooking and made sure everyone had something to drink and eat, and also made sure the older boys were set up with the video game system. When the 12 year old pulled out her math project to finish at our table Tim was there to show her his computer drafting skills. I saw him take an interest in how she was doing. She had to draw a picture to scale copying a smaller picture and complained she was not good at drawing. He was so kind. He took care of most everything today; it was a huge weight off of me. It is clear he does know how hard this is on me.

After they left, I did indulge in a nap. I watched a movie I was unimpressed with and fell asleep. I am hoping the tiredness, cramping, heartburn and emotions are just a part of phase one of pregnancy. A few more days and we find out.

Lying there though, I was convinced I was not pregnant. I really don't feel it—logically I know I should not feel anything. I also know that, just because I don't feel it, doesn't mean it isn't happening inside of me.

I don't know yet. That is that.

February 14, 2011

The sun is shining, the wind is quite pronounced and the blue sky was begging for me to take Bailey for an afternoon walk. I took advantage of natures' windy music and left the headphones at home. I took the time to breathe and relax.

I have a sinking feeling that I am not pregnant. I tend to hope for the best, but expect the worst. I have a safety net that if we are not pregnant and I want to stay home from work and cry, I may tell them my car will not start. I do not want a back-up plan, but I have one. This does not give me rest, it makes me feel guilty. I want to expect the best. I want to be expecting.

Can I turn this negativity around?

I have done all that I was asked to do. I sought medical assistance. I gave blood for repeated tests, and smiled. I asked questions. I was kind. I learned. I read. I prayed. I paid. I called. I had an MRI. I received bad news. I emailed. I worked. I relaxed. I talked. I listened. I administered over 40 shots to myself. I punctually take all medications and vitamins. I gave up alcohol, caffeine and running. I expect my efforts to bring forth greatness. Maybe that greatness is my baby or babies, or maybe that greatness is the space I create to grow into a better woman. Whichever it is, may I graciously accept it as perfect.

February 15, 2011

One day more. (Feel free to belt that out if you are a *Les Misérables* fan.)

Last night in an effort to calm myself, I read one of my (many) yoga magazines that have been piling up. Because I got so into running, I was not keeping up on reading them. Anyway, I read a meditation about sending love to yourself and others. Wishing others happiness, safe from harm or free from suffering. I had sent happiness to one of my sisters, within minutes my phone alerted me to a Facebook posting she just made on my wall. She had shown a picture of me and a stingray to her son who loves aquatic life. To me, it confirmed that at that moment she was experiencing happiness.

I sent joyful thoughts to everyone I could think of and forgot Tim! When I began to think love for him, I realized I really wanted the same for me as for him. I meditated more for him. He came home from work a bit later, with flowers for me. Last night we had talked about not doing anything because, well, we are a bit overwhelmed right now, and yes, I did want flowers for Valentine's, but I want to be pregnant more, so I agreed. And, yet there he was, with flowers for me. They weren't extravagant or even elegant, but he made an effort to make me smile. And it did.

This early morning before getting out of bed I did the meditation again, sending peace and happiness to my embryos, family and friends. I can use all the peace I can get in this stressful time, which honestly, has not been as awful as some other experiences I have had. I will get through this.

I told Tim my fears. Basically, no matter what, we are still one day closer. Either we are pregnant, or we are not and will begin the next plan having learned many lessons. I will be comfortable with the medications, I will be more confident, and I will be more active in taking care of my spiritual and mental health. But, if we are pregnant, I also need to be more active in taking care of my spiritual and mental health…

I have done all that I can do, with what I know and who I am today.

I admit I let my emotions and negative thoughts run away from me. I admit I cried today. I admit that I have no idea how to effectively move through this stress.

Worrying about tomorrow is unfair to you today. I thought this gem up today on my commute home, in tears. Yes, this is so difficult. But I know that I have no idea what tomorrow will bring. Tonight is time to be my own best friend. What would *Tricky* tell me, knowing what test is happening tomorrow?

Girlfriend, we are going to get home from work, eat some nachos maybe ice cream and drink some juice out of a wine glass! We are going to laugh at a funny movie, or watch some trash TV, or quietly read and go to bed. But we will not stay up all night worrying and crying over something we know nothing about. Girl, you are pregnant unless told otherwise. You need to eat, stay hydrated and get some rest. You have an early appointment, and you need to take care of yourself!

I believe that is what she would say to me.

Well, I have had some nachos and some fruit juice in a wine glass. It is late, and I will be heading to bed. I don't know what tomorrow will bring. But, no matter what the test results are, we are still one day closer.

Worrying about tomorrow is unfair to you today.

February 16, 2011

It is the day of our pregnancy test. The most important blood draw of all. It is done quickly, and I leave.

At home I am waiting for the phone call. I admit, I am nervous, anxious and feel like I am on a teeter totter with a fat kid. I am stuck. But, while in the air, I should take a moment to look around.

In the past six months I went to a fertility clinic thinking I knew everything only to learn that inside my body were so many details I could have never imagined. So many things were going wrong and their sole symptom was that I could not get pregnant. In that time frame I learned how far my bravery can get me. I learned that my bravery is not the absence of tears as traditionally thought, but the presence of tears. How in those sad moments I have sought help. I talk to my husband, honestly and openly. I share my intense and embarrassing feelings with him and learned that he does not judge me. I have leaned on my mom, dad, sisters and brothers. I have leaned on friends and been supported. I feel everyone around me cheering these embryos on, and I too, am fiercely rooting for them.

I would be a total liar if I said I was cool and calm waiting for this phone call. But, thankfully I am not a total mess. I have to go to work this afternoon, and I would love to be able to call out—but I know that is not the responsible thing to do. When did I ever say I was responsible?

I know that I am loved. It helps me to repeat that, to reassure myself that I am worth the trouble.

The phone rang, it was an unknown number and I answer it anyway. Though my case nurse was off today, she called me from home to tell me the news. I could hear her smile. *I am pregnant.*

My beta number (the test is referred to as the beta hCG test) was 180, they normally look for between 50 and 100. It will double every two to three days. I have another blood test on Friday, then another most likely on Monday. They will monitor until I get to 2000, then, they will do an ultrasound.

We scream together on the phone as if we are old college roommates sharing and catching up with each other. She went through this with me, I hear her genuine joy, elated for me.

I am amazed. Implantation occurred. It happened. I am euphoric, but with a sigh of relief and humble gratitude. I am stunned and cannot believe that we are here. I know that anything can happen, and that I can have a miscarriage. But, I don't want to worry today. Today, now, I am happy. I am pleased to have received good news. I feel anew. I feel that the world is a bit kinder today. I feel myself exhale, as if I haven't breathed in months.

So, of course I look up my beta number, and the internet told me that a high beta number can mean a miscalculation of conception—not likely, we know the hour sperm was introduced. Or a molar pregnancy—and I made the mistake of reading what that was and now regret it (basically it is not a pregnancy at all, a placenta but no embryo). Or it can be a multiple pregnancy, which is very likely. Keep the positive thoughts flowing, now is not the time to worry, question or wonder. I need to stop Googling.

Days have passed and I am still pregnant! My beta numbers have gone, in a week, 180, 431, 1310 and today 2667. This means that my first ultrasound, of three, will be Monday. We can expect to see a sack (or two) and the main purpose of this is to make sure the embryo sac is in the right place in the uterus. I did not ask, *what if it isn't?* I don't want to think about that answer or possibility. I am still amazed. I have been trusted with a gift.

February 28, 2011

We saw you! One little black oval! You are perfect! I had no idea I could be in love with a black oval.

Forgiveness.

I am pregnant and I am in need of doing a little forgiving. I am in
a constant struggle to forgive myself. I am hard on me. I expect
great things, but in the same breath I expect that it is everyone
else's fault. I have played the victim and martyr and I would like
to look away from that. It is not about imagining what I am
capable of, but actually living through and seeing what I can
accomplish if I get out of my own way. I have let my ego and
insecurity cling to me like a dryer sheet in my sleeve. I have
tolerated the way others treat me, I have allowed myself to be
second. I claim to *run my own race*, but it has not been on a daily
basis. But, I can start, wherever I am.

Is forgiveness about seeking the truth, accepting it and moving
on? Or is it simply about skipping right to the moving on part? I
have a hard time with both; forgiving quickly and easily has never
been my strongest trait. But, what do you gain by holding on to
the hurt? What can I gain by letting it all go? Would I have an
easier time loving? How can I pass the trait of forgiveness on
while simultaneously trying to forge it myself?

I forgive my body. I forgive my pituitary adenoma. I forgive my
spirit, soul and mind that went to dark places. I forgive the over
forty injections. I forgive my work meetings. I forgive the
multiple blood draws and bruises they provided. I forgive my
breasts for being tender. I forgive my abdomen for cramps. I
forgive myself of the worry, tears and pain. I forgive my brain
for wanting to research too much. I forgive myself for making
running priority zero. I forgive myself for thinking too much and
too long on something that hasn't happened and may never
happen. I forgive my past. I forgive my anger, jealousy and self
pity.

I forgive Tim for getting to be the guy in all this. I forgive Tim
for still trying to quit smoking. I forgive Tim for not knowing the
best thing to do or say to me. I forgive Tim for being new to all
of this. I forgive those who I felt did not hurt as much as I did. I

forgive others who were blissfully pregnant. I forgive others who
expressed joy or complaints in their pregnancies. I forgive those
who spoke not knowing what my situation was. I forgive others
for not knowing what to say, for not understanding, for not
comprehending. I forgive others for not asking. I forgive others
for wondering. I forgive myself, and I will keep forgiving
myself. Tomorrow is a new day, may my bucket of forgiveness
be replenished for whatever antics I commit then.

Through this forgiving process, I find myself still holding on to
anger and jealousy; the *why me* part of this whole process. In my
brain I want to stand up for myself, defend my post and proclaim
to the world how hard this has been. I want every naturally
pregnant woman to know, and I want every stereotypical mother-
in-law to know the damage they can do when posing the innocent
question: *When are you going to give me grandchildren*? I feel
the need to shoulder this responsibility, when in reality what my
baby needs is a calm, nurturing place to grow. The fighting needs
to wait, or maybe never come to pass.

I have spent a lot of time fighting, because I felt I have had no
one stand up for me. I want to be heard, I want others to see how
I see it. Unfortunately, I believe I am right. Hasn't this whole
process taught me that I do not know what someone else is going
through? Haven't I learned that you don't always get what you
want? Haven't I learned the positive outcomes that arise when
you simply ask for help?

I cannot let go of these lessons simply because I am now
pregnant. All of this work would then be a sham. How do I hold
on to this? How do I forgive daily? How do I find peace daily?
What reminder do I need that what is important is the little black
oval inside me, thirsty for nutrition, yearning for the safe, warm,
fluffy house I have built. I am living for them, but I need to
maintain me to be successful.

Forgiveness is not tolerance. Forgiveness is acceptance that what
happened, happened, but in the past and there is nothing that can

be done, now, to fix it. Forgiveness is to find peace within the present circumstance. How lucky are we to live another day?

How can I possibly tap into this peace? I have had positive experiences that I can recall upon to ease me. I remember standing in the cool, clear ocean waters as a sting ray glided past my feet. I remember the striking trees in Key West. I remember the calm I felt walking through the Baltimore aquarium with my friend. I remember watching the orangutans at the National Zoo during feeding time with Tim. I remember Tim's face after my embryo transfer when the nurse said, *until your test, you are pregnant.* I remember seeing our house for the first time and the dumbfounded joy when we realized we could afford it. I love when the daffodils come up in spring along the highway of my commute. When someone does something nice for me, like hold a door or say bless you. And now, knowing that soon, within months, I will be a mommy. Can I be determined, each day, to find the good and the things I am grateful for in this world? Can this process continue to make me a better person? Can I keep my mind focused on what is truly important?

I hold a lot of anger and regret in this precious body. I am unfair to others and myself. I am hurt that I had to go through in vitro fertilization. I am hurt because I feel I have been through a lot in my life, and I want something to come easy to me. I judge those who have not been through this, and think that they have it so easy, and I know that I am being unfair, judgmental and harsh. I have no idea what someone else has been through. Their path was no easier than mine. They are no more deserving of gifts than I am. I am no stronger or better than they are. That anger, jealousy and judgment is simply my own insecurity trying to get some attention.

I complain a lot. I think I complain so others will understand and do something about it. When I complain loudest I believe it's because I feel helpless. I think feeling helpless, is one of life's harshest circumstances. I understand logically, that I should only do all that I can, and move on. It is the letting go part that I need to work on.

Here I am, pregnant and angry. The baby needs me to be calm.
The baby needs me to be kind and loving. The baby needs more
than me eating well and resting. I need to create a calm habitat.
A habitat of joy. Through all of this mess, I have forgotten what
brings me joy, I have not allowed the time for things that I enjoy
to come into my life. Here I thought pregnancy would make my
mind calm, as if it were a switch. I have created checklists for
myself. I have neglected the simple pleasures of sitting, listening
to the rain.

I love the rain. I feel the rain has the power to wash away my
tears. I love sleeping in my bed listening to the rain on the roof,
against the windows, tapping the gutters (we have still yet to
clean). I love watching the small rivers wash down the streets
and into the storm drains. I love the power of thunder and
lighting and the pair they make. I love that my whole perspective
on rain changes when I am outside waiting for a bus.

Maybe the answer to *why me* is because I have not yet learned to
be happy wherever I am, and the only way to test me is through
trials. I need to find peace, and I will say it again, start wherever
you are.

I need to re-record the damn record that is on repeat in my head.
The one that thinks I am not good enough, the one that believes
nothing good will happen to me, the one that believes the
negative, the one that slumps her shoulders and cries at night.

Brush off the gravel and finish the race; finish without regrets.
Finish smiling.

As I am now officially pregnant, feeling the glow and the happiness, I know that the world will soon know my secret. It will be protruding out and I face the decision to not only announce my pregnancy but also how I got here. I am proud to be expecting an IVF baby. I am not ashamed, but having harbored this secret for so long, I feel the need to shout it out—so that people will think before they ask dumb, assuming questions into your conception life. I want to be the loudest cheerleader for all my infertility sisters. No one can write this, quite like I can.

A comment on the *Test Tube Baby*: I find the phrase offensive and demeaning to the struggle I endured. It is also inaccurate, but I guess petri dish baby was hard to market. My husband and I pulled the goalie four years before our first visit to an infertility clinic. At this moment, I had a total of 29 doctor's appointments, 20 blood draws, 9 vaginal ultrasounds, 1 dye test, 1 mock embryo transfer, 1 fluid sonogram, 40 self administered subcutaneous injections, 1 intramuscular injection, 1 pill once a day, 1 pill twice a day and 1 vaginal insert three times a day, 1 very important vitamin once a day, 1 cyst drained without anesthesia, 1 MRI where they found an one millimeter adenoma, 1 surgical retrieval of five follicles, 1 transfer of two embryos, 12 days of waiting for a positive blood test, 1 egg sack seen on the ultrasound monitor. 2 sighs of relief, elation and peace from me and my husband. All this, for only 1 IVF cycle; there are countless women who go through this multiple times. Don't you dare demean this trial.

You never know what someone else is going through.

ACT II

Wonder.

Every cramp, twinge of pain or moment of being pain free I wonder; is everything okay, is this normal, am I going to miscarry? In my heart I know all this worry is of no use. It will not make pain go away, it will not manifest a written sign telling me exactly what I want to know. Most of all, reading every book and symptom checker I can about pregnancy will only exacerbate my delicate state.

I am pregnant. Until something horrid happens, I am pregnant. I have been through one of sciences' greatest accomplishments and I had found this process and pregnancy, a gift. I can now look at a child and not cry. I know where I have been, and I know that I have no control over tomorrow.

I have not experienced the nausea yet. I am two days from being 6 weeks, so I am bracing myself. I find myself to be hungry all the time. I have been making healthy snacking choices though, fruit or almonds. I also find myself putting cinnamon on my ice cream—this I have never done before. This is along the other things I am feeling; my body is not my own. I get winded on a few flights of stairs and a mere four months ago I ran a marathon. My knees feel like a robot's knees; I can feel the intricate parts moving together, I walk slow, gingerly manipulating them. My breasts are tender, and I have been wearing only sports bras since back when I was doing the shots. (Ha, remember when *doing shots* was fun?) My breast skin is also tender and even the thought of an underwire cup cutting into me makes my nose wrinkle in disgust. I am more tired than I remember being before. I pee all the time, which interrupts my sleeping time. The progesterone I am on is a vaginal insert and it has a tendency to leak out. I am constantly changing my light days pads. Weird, with all the infertility testing, spotting and now medicinal leaking, I have worn more pads during this process than I have worn for my periods.

Though my belly is not grown, it is bloated. I have been wearing the same pair of jeans to work for two months, I cannot drag myself to getting new clothes just yet, I feel like that would be a waste. I am very sensitive to what is going on inside of there. So much so that I cautiously sleep on my side and find myself thinking, oh, I should not twist my body like that, what if the cord snaps off from my lining and the embryo drifts helplessly down my uterine water slide?

Pregnant woman should get to have the whole gestation time off from work, and get a year of maternity leave too. I know we fought for women's' liberation and we still are fighting for equal wages; but seriously, why are we adding so much more stress to our lives when the creation and growth of a new person is way more important than another meeting on how to properly fill out a timesheet.

I do find that it is easier to focus at work now that I am pregnant. The waiting, stress, shots and monitoring appointments during the IVF cycle were far more debilitating for me. However, now I am super careful with myself in my active job, I am way more snarky towards ignorant colleagues and I am more apt to taking time off when I feel I need it.

My home is dirtier. Okay, not dirty in the hoarding sense, but not the way I used to keep it.

I discover everything you eat, crave or do is bad for the baby. Look it up online, you will be paralyzed with fear at every entry. Also, once the baby finally arrives, everything in your home will cause SIDS.

They gave me your first picture. You look like a black oval on a landscape of grey and white. I put it on the fridge. I know I will frame it, and the ones to follow too. I thought about keeping it in my purse, but if it is on the fridge so your daddy can see it too, whenever he needs to. He is quitting smoking today, you are his inspiration; he has been trying for a very long time. We both

One egg sack. I did grieve a little for the embryo that was
transferred that we did not see on the screen. I was a bit
disappointed that there was not more than one, only because we
do want more than one child and I did not want to go through the
IVF process again. Then, in the same breath:

*I was so proud of you for surviving! You are so strong. You were
out of five follicles and you were the one that made it! This just
cements the idea that you can do anything you want in life and
your dad and I will be your biggest supporters.*

March 10, 2011

*Today, we saw your heart beating! It looked like a flashing grain
of white rice. 143 beats a minute, which concerned your daddy!
He did not yet know that your pulse is completely normal and
perfect! It nearly gave him a heart attack, until our physician's
assistant let him know that it was all fine, and we were right on
target. I am seven weeks pregnant with you, and the nausea and
vomiting has started.*

The morning sickness is not as awful as I thought it would be, for
me. I am lucky. For some reason, it is more socially accepted to
throw up, well, pretty much anywhere, whereas diarrhea, you
really need a toilet or a tree. Public defecation is frowned upon
and gross whereas public vomit—eh, that's cool.

*They gave us another picture of you, this time we can see you a
bit better. You are a white and grey pixilated mass, and we love
you. I put it on the fridge.*

Blessings.

I got a message from my sister last night, she is two years older than me and a mother of two. She is currently 14 weeks pregnant, me 8 weeks. My instinct was joy for her and happy that we would be pregnant together though we live in different states.

Then later my demons kicked in. The jealous voice in my head thinking silly, ridiculous thoughts.   What if she has picked the same names Tim and I have dreamed about for years?   She is further along, she will win. Who will my mom stay with after delivery, we are only weeks apart and my parents are in their 70's; I want my mom to be with me after the baby is born. These silly thoughts panicked me.

My logical brain knew this was all silly. My heart also realized, that she knew she was pregnant while I was going through my IVF cycle—and she was happy for me. She asked how I was feeling, she was concerned. She showed me grace by waiting to tell me until I at least knew we had a heartbeat. I also learned through my mom, that her pregnancy is partially my fault. While I was seeking fertility treatments she told me she would give me her eggs if needed. I wept when she told me this; what a gift. Well, apparently she had taken herself off her birth control pill in case I would ask her to help us. Sometimes, when we try to bless others, we get blessed ourselves.

Another lesson for me; listen to your heart—that is your true self, your brain is the secretary, don't get them confused and give the assistant more responsibility than it can handle.

Typical.

I opened the fridge scouting out dinner and saw raw chicken. My stomach turned, I wretched and headed to the bathroom. I stood there a bit, realizing I would not be eating chicken for dinner—at least I would not be the one responsible for cooking it. I vomited, it splashed up into my hair and I resigned myself that instead of making dinner I would be taking a shower.

Tim left the house to get me ginger ale.

Morning sickness, it turns out, is any time of day. I keep crystallized ginger and small snacks handy. For me, if I wasn't hungry, I was nauseous. And, I would actually throw up—there are old wives tales telling the sex of the baby based on whether or not you actually throw up; girl if you did, boy if you didn't.

I have amazing dreams while pregnant, with soundtracks, large plot lines and colorful characters. I also begin to eat a lot of pickles and mayonnaise; together…it is delicious...

Coming out.

I have been waiting to tell people we were pregnant. In my head I want to wait until after the first trimester. Another part of me just wants to gloss over it, and another part would rather tell perfect strangers than co-workers.

My boss asked for when I wanted leave for the next year, we are working out our vacation schedule. So, I felt that he needed to know, and my two immediate co-workers already knew because I needed help from them covering my shifts when I had the egg retrieval and transfer. My sisters and parents knew, because how do you go through this without them?

How do you tell your world? I feel that the IVF part of the story is crucial. I feel like not mentioning it takes away how special this is. It diminishes how hard we worked for it; how awful life was. I feel like ignoring it, ignores the patience, tears, shots, appointments, more tears, and all the pain I experienced even before I get to labor. I feel like I have earned a spot on a podium for an extra-special *atta girl*! I want other ladies dealing with infertility to know they have a friend in me. I want to be their advocate. I want infertility normalized. Why don't we talk about this—why haven't I?

Our immediate families knew; you can't let the people who have been on the journey with you, left hanging after the two week wait. I was on spring break from work, so not making an official announcement was preferable; I had rather the information trickle down.

Then, we told Facebook at 10 weeks. I wasn't totally comfortable with it, I wanted to wait longer, but at this time we felt like we could handle it, whatever that meant.

Tim posted our most recent ultrasound with text that said, *HEY! We've got a baby coming! And now I'm that guy that posted the ultrasound picture on Facebook.*

I let everyone know that with the help of IVF we would be expecting in October.

Quickly and prolifically, the private messages began to flood my inbox. It usually started off with, *we have been trying for X number of years…*

My mission begins. Infertility and miscarriages are silent, lonely battles. Unnecessarily silent battles. With each message there was one of my friends isolated and tragically sad. All of the same feelings I too had hid, they had too. The shame, the fear, anger, jealousy all of it—shared experience with all of these women and together we had no idea we were not alone.

Passing the baton.

We are released from the care of our infertility specialists after ten weeks and begin our pregnancy journey they way normal women do; by seeing an OB/GYN. As instructed by my fertility center, I make an appointment with an OB/GYN upon a recommendation from our doctors. I call when I am eight weeks, before our final ultrasound with our IVF doctors, expecting we will be released to a *normal baby doctor's* care soon.

At our final IVF appointment, they called it our graduation; we saw another glimpse at our little one. We saw *her* move. Since I first saw the little yolk sack, I decided I was having a girl. Well, we saw the head, an ear, fingers, and she did a little turn. It was remarkable. When she moved, Tim, said, *holy shit!* It was amazing for us all. We were told that everything was good and normal; we were led to another room—the same room that only months ago we started this discussion. We were given paperwork and sent on our way. I was asked that I visit them so they can see me pregnant, and they wanted an email once she was born, they want to know who this little person is. So do I. Normal felt unreal.

Ten days after our third ultrasound we are waiting in a room one floor above the fertility clinic. It is a smaller waiting room, happy, with photos of pregnant women and babies on the walls. It is approaching Easter, so plastic eggs and spring flowers are on the receptionist's window. As we wait I fill out what is necessary and I am armed with my paperwork and a notebook of questions. I am ready to be informed. We wait with women who are visibly pregnant and men who look uncomfortable in these surroundings. I sit happily, I am where I want to be; Tim is content checking his phone and sharing with me the humorous sports related commentary he is reading.

I am asked to urinate into a paper cup. Being the overachiever I had a situation of overflow. I dump out some and leave what I think is an adequate and acceptable amount. Then wash my hands…three times.

We get called back into an exam room, Tim goes with me. We are greeted by a nurse with a neck tattoo and a gold tooth. She takes my weight and blood pressure. The nurse notices my notebook and brings me a pregnancy journal that a sales rep gives them. It has an area for my questions, appointments and a place for my pictures. It makes me feel like a normal, cutesy, Pinterest, pregnant woman. I am elated. This truly makes me feel whole. It is not a place to log injections, results, numbers, acronyms, questions and follow up appointment and tests…it is a log for joy.

Our doctor comes in, she is a boisterous woman. It is hard to read her age. She sits down and asks me several questions. She asks about the Celiac and the Hashimoto's disease and proceeds to tell us about a twenty-eight mile bike ride she did with her son. She tells us that she pooped out at the end and rode back in the truck with an old hippy man with long grey hair. He was interested in starting a gluten free bakery. Our doctor added that she had a hunch some of his products would have marijuana in them, and *that would be fine*. We talk a bit more about why I needed IVF, and she seemed like she knew what she was talking about and confident. She left the room for me to undress for an exam.

She returned and joked about Tim still being with me; "usually the guys head for the hills for the pelvic exam!"

"Tim has been at most of my appointments." I explain.

"I bet you could administer the transvaginal ultrasound!" she said.

"Probably, I would at least know what to be looking for." He jokes.

The pelvic exam is quick. I am told to get dressed and head to her office where we will finish the appointment. It feels like just another day for her.

Her office is angular, the corner office of a strangely shaped building. Some of the photos and certificates are askew, and though it is not cluttered, there is a lot in her office. A particular family photo steals my attention. It looks like there is a cut out picture over what would be the husband in the family portrait. I point it out to Tim, he stands up to get a closer look he thinks it is James Taylor. Sure enough, he looks it up on his phone and it is a photo of him from the album, *Sweet Baby James*. We wanted to ask her about it, but the first appointment seemed like the wrong time.

She enters her office and gives her well rehearsed newly pregnant patient welcome speech. We are a little over ten weeks and she goes over the ins and outs of nutrition, recommended vitamins, testing options and calming me down.   She then tells me how ahead of the game I am with my gluten free diet and not too be too worried,

"Heroin addicts often have healthy babies!" she exclaims.

She then acknowledges that we are parents in a *premium pregnancy*, we have been through a lot with infertility and now it is her job to scrape us off the ceiling and have a healthy baby. She tells me I can run, and even rock climb if I wanted to. She says that she would never tell me that something I did caused a miscarriage. Crazy as she seems, she is a perfect fit for us. In the same appointment she mentioned pot, heroin and that she will never blame me for a miscarriage. She checked all the boxes for the OB I need in my life right now.

Though I am a grateful expecting lady, I have taken to blaming the baby for things I do. For instance, the baby often forgets to run the dishwasher, fold the laundry or send a particular email. The baby also voices her appetite; *the baby wants three eggs for dinner*. The baby loves gluten free chocolate cake. The baby also causes my nausea, painful boobs and outright forgetfulness. It is a joyous and fun loving way of teasing me via the impending baby, and it helps me remember that it is real. We are pregnant. I did have a positive beta test. We did see it on an ultrasound. My symptoms are real. I do not have my period.

April 26, 2011

Yesterday was my 32nd birthday. I am 32, pregnant, with a home and a loving husband—it is wonderful! I took time off, and it was the Easter holiday so it all worked out; I was able to see family and rest. Though, lately, no rest has ever been enough.

I am in my 14th week, there are times I can't believe I am pregnant. Every time I pee and don't see period I am so happy and relieved.

My pants don't quite fit, but through the generosity of four sisters and friends I have maternity clothes to wear. I am very grateful for these hand-me-downs; turns out, the world of motherhood is a very kind place. Interesting how the world of *trying to get pregnant* is not.

Tim and I are both nesting. Cleaning up the house, getting organized, crossing to do items off the list and of course, getting excited.

He awoke with a nightmare the other morning, a sense of evil foreboding. I was awake too, but I shared with him that I had a dream about our little girl and she loves the water—that we had to pull her out of my sister's pool and she was crying because she wanted to stay in longer! She loves swimming. This made Tim smile and he was able to go back to sleep. I am glad we can work together like that.

Work stress is still plaguing me. That is my evil foreboding. Tim has been trying to figure out how much of a take home salary and insurance he would need to bring home in order to allow for me to stay at home. And, who knows if I want that. I think I do, but I have never been a full time mom. It is a lot to think about. What I question though is, I have a degree—Tim does not, who really should be the one to be in the workforce? What are our best chances? Every job is going to cause me stress—and Tim historically has an easier time leaving work at work. But, do you ask your partner to take on the whole load? How do we share this? How do we each do our part to support each other? We can talk about it all we want, but the truth is, the baby is not here yet and there is so much left unknown.

We will keep talking, that I know. It is our only possibility towards a solution.

Who will you be?

I cannot wait to meet you—but I will wait until you are healthy enough to survive outside my body. We chose your name possibilities (though the boy name, I am not completely sold on…) based on a name that would help you do anything or be anybody you want to be.

We loved you when you were a follicle, and each day I continue to nurture that love. I am also working on my mom guilt—I had a bunch of salty and sugary food last night and I just felt so bad for you! Each week that marks your existence we read what size you are and how your little body is developing. I tell your daddy, our baby is an onion! We both get excited.

We joke about what kind of person you will be. Because your dad and I think that we are funny, we tease that you will be a very serious and literal person. Transversely, we tease that we are in so much trouble because you are going to be our personality and traits multiplied!

We wonder what you will look like, brown hair, red hair, blonde? Who will you resemble more? What your birth date will be and how labor will go.

Next week we get to find out if you are a boy or a girl; we joke that you will make it difficult and hide your parts from us causing us another surprise in all of this! Again, we love you, no matter what.

May 18, 2011

More and more, couples are coming out of the woodwork sharing that they have infertility or think they do. I feel a distinct need, almost like a gravitational pull to help, listen and share with them what I have learned and lived. So far all are appreciative, and I think the current baby bump offers them hope.

This new role also offers me hope; a purpose that everything means something. That I truly can be a positive person, that I can have a spirit that helps others.

Whoa.

We head to our appointment, the sonogram to tell us that the baby is healthy and okay and, if she cooperates we learn what the gender is. I told Tim in the kitchen that I think she is a girl, and I will think that until I am told otherwise.

We wait. The technician has called out sick and they are sending someone else over to do the sonogram but we need to wait a little longer. I use the restroom while we continue to wait.

Tim jokes and says,

"You know, I am good with tools…a sonogram is kind of like a stud finder, right? How about I just do it?" I am the only one who laughs. (I think this is his first dad joke.)

Our technician arrives, apologizes, and asks if we want to know the sex of the baby, we quickly respond *yes* as I hop onto the butcher paper.   I am asked to lift my shirt and pull my pants and underwear down a bit lower. The warm, blue goo is squeezed on my belly and she begins the sonogram. She exclaims that right away our little one has displayed herself! It is unmistakably a little girl—though to me it is a grey, white and black mass! Apparently our little one was bent over to display her gender. Tim's hair turned grey right then and there.

Then we saw her kicking and punching all over the place, she was extremely active and funny. Each time the technician tried to get a certain measurement she would move and do something to prevent her from getting all of her data. At one point we saw her with ankles crossed, and hands behind her head, as if she was chillin' in a pool!

It was a marvelous experience, to see her so happy and healthy and average. It was as if she was saying to us, *I got this, stop worrying about me, I am having fun…backstroke…*

The awe that came over us was delicious. It was normal. It was problem-free. It was weird…

We told everyone about her, announced that she was a *she* and exclaimed about how every measurement meant that she was healthy and strong. We started to call her by the name we picked out, and love referring to her as *she* and *her room* and when *she gets here*; it is bliss. The joy in Tim's eyes upon knowing that she was a she and doing okay, was beautiful. Her existence has made him softer, and a better man. Me? Well, I am still working on me…

After a run I showered. (Remember Dr. Pot Heroin said I could run now.) While leaning over to towel dry my hair I felt something. Like the wing of a butterfly flapping against my abdomen from the inside. I stood still, frozen. I felt it again. I felt it a few more times, got dressed and told Tim,

"I think I felt something!"

Not knowing exactly what the feeling of feeling life was, it was difficult to determine if I had indeed felt life. Knowing that she moved around so much during the ultrasound made me wonder.

The butterfly wing feeling happened again after another run, and I was pretty sure it was her. Then one night while lying in bed I was sure. I ran down stairs, and told Tim to come to bed. I lay down, I put his hands on my abdomen and within a minute we both felt a BA BOOM punch.

We glowed, Tim said, "That was her!"

Each day I make sure that I feel her; mostly it is when I am sitting or lying down, but recently, in week 22, I feel her all the time. She has now seemed to settle in the center of my abdomen, I feel a lot of the movement on the sides of the belly button region.

When you read about the feeling of life it is described as butterflies in your stomach or even gas. For me it was at first a wing, then quick hits. Now it is kicks and rolls, as though she is whooshing around in the amniotic fluid.

June 30, 2011

I simply love you, little one.

I love her. I love feeling her life and her joy. But I am having a hard time soaking it all in. I allow the stress of my work to consume me. Here, this little fighter is being nourished by me— and only me, and I am stressing about work? How fair is that?

I am the only one who can carry her, who can help her live and grow. It is my responsibility to nourish her, to rest, to hydrate and to seek peace. No one is going to do it for us. But this is not and should not be considered a burden. This is a gift. I worked for this gift, and I deserve to experience every moment of this treasure. To savor the kicks, the weight gain, the leg cramps, the breathlessness, the uncomfortable sleep, the anxiety of giving birth, the overwhelming amount of stuff we need for her, getting the house ready for her arrival, eating, and glowing. All of it is included in the benefits package to the job of becoming a mother. I fought for this job, I played by the rules and I know I am qualified. I know I am capable of great joy, peace and happiness. I know I can do this. I simply need to remember to breathe through it all and enjoy the race.

Most nights when we are in bed trying to fall asleep Tim will rest his hand on my belly, for this is when my little girl is most active. There is such joy for us, simply feeling her life. I never could have dreamed this wonder for us.

She is so very strong and when she gives big kicks Tim says,

"Whoa, there she is!"

Who needs sleep?

I know, I know, once the baby arrives a mommy will never sleep
again. I understand that is coming, but now, since the second
trimester I have not had a full night's rest. Why? Because my
little wonder is a dancer.

Sometimes it is hip hop, sometimes a groovy wave like jive but
whenever I lay down, or even sit to rest with my feet up she goes
to town! I have concerns. First, since there is all this dancing
while I am trying to sleep, I am not getting enough rest and I feel
depleted and worn out. Second, does this mean that when she
comes out she will only sleep when being rocked and moved
around, like she does in the womb? Will I ever rest again?

To be clear, my body has also decided that I need to wake up
every three hours—which is as if my body is preparing itself for
the upcoming feedings. In reality, this is all very cool. How is it
that my body knows what it needs to do right now; after all the
IVF craziness, it is as if my body is now saying, *I got this*. So,
now you want to be an arrogant star student? Thanks, your timing
is terrible.

It all started with the kicking and punching style of dancing; less
grace, more epileptic hippopotamus. And I would wake and have
a hard time getting comfortable with such a strange experience.
Then the leg cramps, which I would hydrate myself more to help
prevent the leg cramps, which leads to the evening pee breaks.
Then the stress and worry over my job, maternity leave, day care,
why can't I quit my job and be a stay at home mommy, all of
which would echo through my head.   Soon it felt like I could not
sit up anymore, as if my stomach muscles had all vanished. All
the discomfort prompted us to by the most expensive, craziest
pillow I never thought I would buy. It is a U shape, $100 bucks,
and man it is worth it. It hugs you, you can maneuver your leg
around it and get all cozy and comfy—and, you can roll over and
do the same thing on the other side. Most pregnancy pillows are

one sided options and you need to roll over and take them with you. I am too lazy to do that, those other ones are shaped like a J.

However, be warned. We have a name for the pillow. *The Celibacy Pillow.* You see, it is so cozy and comfy, I don't want to snuggle with my husband, and the pillow is so huge that it takes up half of our king sized bed. If we do feel like some contact, I open up the celibacy pillow door to let him in. In conclusion, it is helping me…him, not so much.

What is not helping is my stress level. I am now 30 weeks in, and not appreciating all the wonders that is happening inside of me, that I fought so hard to achieve. It is not fair to me, to her, or my husband. I don't want to move through this pregnancy half assed. I went through IVF doing everything possible, being faithful and diligent, why stop that good habit now? Haven't I learned? Do everything possible and you will succeed. I wanted this experience, now that I have it I need to embrace it. Love every moment of it. I am tired, who cares? I am making a person! I have a little girl dancing inside of me, showing me that she is okay and that she is growing and I simply cannot wait to meet her. This pregnancy has gone so fast, and yet trying to get pregnant went by so painstakingly slow.

How can I savor these weeks, this final trimester? What positive light can I shed to see me through this with the presence that is necessary? How best can I train for this mommy marathon? How can I treasure all of this?

Start wherever you are.

This evening I took a bath. It brought me closer to her, there we were both in our own bag of waters. I was reminded that I enjoy swimming, and that maybe going to the pool in this final trimester can provide me some exercise and help ease my joints. I was reminded that all my stressing was actually making my worries more powerful. Here I was giving my stressors all the attention, when in reality the most important thing I have is inside of me,

growing and fighting for my attention. Who is the one who
should win? She should always win. And finally, I remembered
how much I needed this book, to write, to capture all of this. To
remind myself of my *Tricky Cervix*, where I have been and where
I am headed.

I have everything I need. I simply need to accept it. To welcome
it into my life. Whatever you feed is what will grow, I need to
stop feeding my anxiety, worry and stress and start feeding peace,
joy and hope.

At week 35 I had the hospital bag packed. It was a like an
overnight bag if I were going somewhere and never would see the
public. Solely comfort items, toiletries, comfy clothes and *her*
going home outfit. The bag is in the car waiting for our trip. We
were also instructed to get flu shots—my first ever flu shot. At
this time we also selected our pediatrician, a parent friend of ours
recommended a group; Tim went to the open house and was
thrilled with them. I checked out their web site and loved the
information, everything about them and the fact that one of the
doctors has Celiac. Also, it is less than two miles from our home.
The pediatrician and my OB were the ones suggesting the flu
shot. We will be bringing a baby into the world at the peak of flu
season, it is best to protect her. Tim also had to get TDAP which
also is the vaccine for whooping cough, which has recently made
a comeback. Apparently I get that shot when leaving the hospital.

We are at 36 weeks, I feel huge and dare I say it, uncomfortable.
I cannot wait to greet this baby and all the while I know that I
wanted this pregnancy so bad—I think I thought it would make
me a better person somehow. But I realize that putting so much
stock in the *if only I had…* does not do me any good.

I have strayed from prayer and positive thinking this last
trimester. I have been so tired that I am not quite sure who I am
anymore. I know that the identity crisis will only strengthen
when she is born, after all, I will be a mommy first—then who
else next…

I have strayed from writing as well. Forgetting what was important and how I got here. I have been working a lot; including long days—in which I do not get compensated for. (Fun fact, I discuss with HR where I may be able to pump at work, the response was a blank stare…) I have been extremely hesitant to take any sick days, because after she is born, I will want as much time off as possible. But today, I am too tired. Last night I believe I was having Braxton Hicks contractions. No rhythm to them, but a pain like period cramps and my abdomen was all hard. Tim is away on a work training trip for two days, and of course I am worried—so that doesn't help anything. So, I took a gamble and chose to stay home from work today. I slept a good part of the morning, and my plan is to take it easy and take care of myself. We shall see how that goes.

At my next appointment our due date was moved up, I was 50 percent effaced, so this means my cervix has thinned. This is measured by the highly technological method of Dr. Pot Heroin physically examining my vagina with her hands. I have no other reason to doubt her, so I take this as a sign that delivery is close, so once I arrive to work I hand over shows to coworkers and asked my manager that I be put on *office duty* instead of actively coordinating the production aspects of performances. No one questions this.

At my next OB appointment we get a sonogram and learned that she is breech. She is butt down, head up.

What? All of the sudden I went from thinking about pain management, breathing and a natural childbirth to the very likely possibility of a cesarean section. I went home and cried.

Of all the childbirth and rearing classes we went to, we missed the one on cesarean sections. Albeit, we had a good reason, we had an earthquake and I physically felt sick for the rest of the day, so we skipped birthing class that night. So, then, as a nervous pregnant lady is wont to do, I search online about ways to turn the baby around and about c-sections. Quickly though, I decide to surrender; let whatever happen, happen. It is not up to me, this is not a hurdle, this is just a different track. This is one of the first times I can ever recall being at peace with a change of plans. I don't know exactly how I found my way there, but trying to spin a baby seemed like it wasn't meant to be, so I simply stopped reading the information and accepted that we would very likely have a c-section, and that would be okay.

It is October 12, 2011. I am 38 weeks and 6 days.

I woke up with a contraction, as I have the past two mornings. However, then about 20 minutes later I had another one. Before Tim left for work I had six, so I stayed home from work.

I have a well of emotions—never feeling really what a contraction feels like I called my mom. My dad answered and was actually able to talk to me about it—which is not surprising since he is the father of ten kids.

I explain that it feels like waves of menstrual cramps—but I am not feeling like how it is depicted in the movies or TV. I am not screaming or grabbing on to furniture, so what is this?

He tells me that "Yup, that sounds 'bout right!"

While we are talking my mom comes home from the store, my dad tells her it is me on the phone.

She says, "Is she contracting, 'cause this is the weather for it!"

We laugh and say *yes*. We talk a bit more, then hang up.

The weather for contractions is a grey, dreary, rainy day, I write down every contraction time and text it to Tim—as he has asked me to. They continue all day, around 3pm though they are a bit stronger and I start to get nervous. Since she is breech my instructions are that if they go to 8 minutes apart for an hour to call my doctor. They skip the eight minute intervals and jump to five minutes, so I call the office. I get the answering service and nervously tell them what is going on.

My ego jumps into my head. You see, today is my mother in law's birthday. I don't want my baby to share a birth date; I want it to be her own. I sigh, knowing that I will not get what I want, the way I want it, in this life, once again, I learn surrendering.

I am instructed to go to the hospital. Tim is on his way home and I call my parents and let them know we are going to head over. They tell me to call no matter what time it is, and they sound so happy that grandchild number 18 may be arriving shortly.

Tim comes home and is not at all his calm self. He rushes in the house and seems to have a flustered whirlwind approach to life while, though contracting, I am feeling fine and relaxed. I am so calm, I watch him like I would watch someone frantically searching for the eyeglasses they are currently wearing. I tell him I have called my parents and they know we are on the way to the hospital. He tells me his folks would *want that call too*. I take this to mean that he has told them that I have been contracting all day and that birth today was an actual possibility.

We get in the car, it is raining hard and the hospital is about 30 minutes away without traffic. But, it is now 5pm, raining, and in the Baltimore area this means it will take a long time to get there. Oh, and there is also construction everywhere and it seems he manages to hit every pot hole in existence. I am still 5 minutes apart but not feeling any downward pushing at all, simply the feeling of an intense tightening. It feels like I have an elastic band around my abdomen which every five minutes cinches tighter.

He asks me to call his mom. I dial, she picks up, I say hi and she immediately asks if she can call me back.

Astonished that there is something more pressing for her to attend to then me in labor, I respond, "Uh, no, we are on the way to the hospital."

"Oh, what, oh, ok!"

"Yeah, I'll have Tim call you later."

I hang up very confused. Turns out Tim has not spoken to his parents at all today—she thought I was calling to wish her a happy birthday and she was already on the other line with my brother in law. Tim and I crack up about this. I tell him to be sure to explain to her the misunderstanding.

Tim asks me if I packed him pajama pants in the hospital bag. I say yes, and he is relieved he won't meet any doctors or nurses with his dick hanging out. I laugh and then yell at him that you should not make a contracting woman laugh and hit a pothole all at the same time. Boys sure are concerned about their equipment being seen by medical professionals, aren't they? Must be nice to have gone through this all without *your* junk hanging out…

We pass three hospitals on our way to ours. Tim jokes that the hospital signs should say, *If you chose us, you would have had your baby by now.*

We arrive at the labor and delivery building. It has a valet option and a drop off the pregnant lady section. Tim goes into the hospital with me, leaving the car unlocked, keys in ignition and running. (Where are my glasses!) I point this out to him, he ignores me, and the valet attendant gives me a reassuring nod and smile waving that he will watch the car for us. I am sure this is not the first time an expectant dad has left the car on, open and vulnerable in front of the labor and delivery building.

I sign in then pace in the waiting area until I am called into the exam room. I am asked to provide a urine sample and undress. I am hooked up to a belly monitor and I wait. Tim returns from actually parking the car, with our bag, and pillows—that we will not be using because she is breech and we are pretty certain we are going to have a c-section. This time, I ignore him for a bit. I breathe and do whatever I am asked to do. I am told that I am not dilated at all, still breech and contracting *like crazy*. The nurse exits to speak to my OB doctor-who happens to be on call this evening. It is now 12 hours from my first contraction.

The nurse comes back in and says,

"Well, you are going to have your baby tonight."

My doctor has decided to do the c-section immediately rather than making me come back at 12:01am. You see, tonight I am one day shy of 39 weeks. Technically, they cannot perform a c-section unless medically necessary. I am told later that my bag of waters ruptured, though I do not remember that. I kind of feel like this was the OB version of *wink it fell off a truck wink.*

As soon as this decision is made, labor and delivery nurses swarm our tiny exam room. I am being asked questions, shaved, IV set up and asked to sign waivers, all at the same time. There are gloved hands everywhere. Tim decides that now is as good a time as any to get dressed in his scrubs. His nervous excitement is adorable. I feel more calm and at peace than I have ever felt.

The catheter was the worst part. I was told that it was supposed to feel like I had to pee—and it did. It was so annoying, it was probably what kept me grounded in the midst of how fast everything was moving. Years of wanting this, and finally, I would have my baby, but damn it can you let me pee first!

The spinal anesthesia was a non issue for me, my doctor and the anesthetist commented about how *in the zone* I was. For me, it was about breathing in and out. I felt like all the world went away, it was just me, waiting for my little girl. I felt ready. I once again surrendered to what was happening letting go of any attachment I had. I let go. It was the same bliss as when I was told,

"As of right now, you are pregnant."

They help lay me down, Tim is brought in and a blue sheet divider hides my belly. Tim holds my hand and kisses my forehead. I am asked if I feel anything sharp, I don't, I feel a sensation of being touched but nothing specific.

They begin. Then I hear grunting, my doctor is having a hard time getting the baby out—her head (which, is huge) is stuck under my ribs. Tim stands up to peer over the divider and I hear him say, *whoa*, and he is back on his stool. He tells me she is almost here. (When Tim re-tells what he saw, he says that Dr. Pot

Heroin has her foot on the stretcher as leverage pulling our girl out of my war torn, shredded abdomen.) I actually feel an internal tugging and I catch my breath as they move a mirror to show her exit. I simply look, focusing upward, I do not want to see what I look like cut open—why would I want to see my surgically opened self!? But there she is. Grey and filthy with her mouth open in a silent cry. They bring her over to a table and we hear her first cries.

A clichéd single tear escapes my eye as the anesthetist wipes it away for me and tells me that her cry is exactly what they want to hear. It is noted that she was born at 8:01pm, and Tim tells them all her name is Juliet Hope. She then sneezes on her daddy. Tim brings her over to my face and I am in awe.

Once I am stitched up I am moved into the recovery room where I meet back up with Tim and Juliet. I cannot feel my arms or my whole body—which is an awful feeling—so Tim and the nurse help position Juliet so I may breastfeed her. Tim calls our families to announce her arrival. A little 7 pound 12 ounce 20 inch long firecracker, who was worth the wait, has arrived.

We are then moved into a room we will stay for the next few days. From my phone I email my boss and co-workers;

"So…my maternity leave starts today. Juliet Hope Manning arrived at 8:01 pm this evening!"

So, what happens now?

Everything did change. Schedules, priorities, my body—
everything changed. After her birth I seemed to develop dinosaur
scale dandruff, fantastic farts and cravings of nothing but wine
and chocolate. I understand how moms can turn into alcoholic,
overweight women. I did not sleep, I had postpartum depression
and there were days I couldn't figure out what day of the week it
was, even when the morning shows told me.

In the beginning I wrote this because no one knew my story. No
one understood me and my tragic pain. My woe, heartache, and
utter sadness it was mine alone. I wrote this to gain empathy, so
others would understand and maybe they would judge less, think,
then speak, or maybe just care more. I wrote out of a selfish
yearning that someone else would hurt as much as I did. That if
they hurt too, I would be validated, or exist.

Writing this, disarmed me. Discovering the idea of a *Tricky
Cervix* showed me, I do not need to fight so hard. I need to admit
defeat, ask for help and do everything possible to achieve my own
goal. How simple an idea, but how difficult it is to realize. How
many other things in life do we fight to achieve; struggle after
struggle instead of simply opening ourselves up to the idea that
we have no clue what we are doing. We do not know what is
best, we only know what is in our heart and sometimes it takes a
bit longer for the heart to translate to the brain what the next step
is. Spoiler alert, it requires surrender.

I believe my own next step is to make the time, the space in my
life to hear that translation. I believe I need to take time each day
to listen to my heart, in the quiet, and allow myself mistakes
along the way. I do not know what is next, but I must trust that it
will be exactly what I need at that moment in my life. Start,
wherever you are.

I have been told that infertility is an emotional roller coaster. I
disagree. Roller coasters are fun. Infertility is like being on a

community trampoline, but you have fallen. You are awkwardly struggling to get up but everyone else keeps jumping…and they are laughing together, enjoying themselves and have not noticed you are trying to get up, so they keep happily jumping.

I have my little girl. She has her own room and life completely changed in this house. I have been very open that she is an IVF baby, and the number of couples who have come out to say they have been experiencing the same heartache, is overwhelming. So, maybe I also wrote this for everyone else; all the fertile couples. Maybe they can read this and understand a little of what you are going through. However your baby comes into your world, let it know its value to you, let them know they are irreplaceable and live your life understanding that you have no idea what someone else may be going though, so be kind and try to surrender.

ACT III

Babies are hard.

I quit my job and became a full time mom. My resignation letter had spilled breast milk on it; I enjoyed the stereotypical hot mess new mom cliché I became. Another marathon was run, and sentences came out of my mouth I never dreamed of uttering and some things I will never un-see.

It was almost two years after our IVF attempt. Juliet was doing amazing, and we knew we wanted her to have a sibling. I have nine siblings, Tim has two. I feel that growing up with a sibling helps create your character, and no matter what—even after all the fights, stealing of clothes, teasing and living in the shadow of their greatness—your sibling loves you, and would do anything for you. Basically, we wanted to create a teammate for Juliet.

Our plan was to try again the old fashioned way for six months, and then we would go back to the fertility clinic. This was a bit of a stressor for us; we now had different insurance and no fertility treatments would be covered. I was a stay at home mom, Tim was our sole breadwinner. We simply did not have the money for another assisted pregnancy.

I went to my endocrinologist and asked if we could try to get my TSH to a good fertility place and see if that could help our chances. During this we learned that my Hashimoto's became active and my antibody titer was higher than it ever had been. He started me on the thyroid medication once again, and we would have monthly appointments and follow up blood work.

For our first attempt I used an ovulation kit and on the first day of testing, while still menstruating, we got the GO sign. We romped and hoped. I did an early at home pregnancy test and it was negative. My period was then two days late so I tested again, and low and behold we got a positive pregnancy test, I called all my doctors, stopped the post partum depression medication, increased the dose on the thyroid medicine and waited expectantly for our first appointment. For some odd reason, your OB will not see you until you are between 8 to 10 weeks. Why so cavalier? You are making a baby! Why don't you want to monitor me immediately? Apparently, this is what happens to normal couples. I missed the daily monitoring, why doesn't Amazon have at home sonograms?

We began the exciting planning. We were going to move Juliet to the office, and new baby would have her old room. It was so amazing; I felt like I was being blessed for all that we went through, and all the praying for other women I was doing…it was a gift.

At around 7 weeks I started spotting, at 2:30am. I prayed. When morning came I told Tim, and when my OB's office opened, I called and told them what was going on. It was only slight spotting, just when I wiped and it was pink and sometimes brown. They had me come in for an ultrasound that afternoon. The baby measured 6 weeks 3 days and had a heartbeat of 111. I got a picture and was sent home. My doctor's assistant called a few hours later to tell me everything looked normal and just to take it easy and stay hydrated. My scheduled appointment was about 2 weeks away, but I was to call if there were any changes.

The next morning, on Valentine's Day, after Tim left for work I felt a horrible contraction, then a gush between my legs. I went into the bathroom and on my panty liner was bright red blood. I felt another whoosh and the feeling of leaking. I saw in the toilet a large clot. It looked like an egg yolk only dark red almost black. I stayed there a short period of time, once I felt I was done draining I cleaned up and tried to call the doctor's office, it was not yet open. A few more gushes happened and about two hours later I was feeling a bit better, the pain had slowed. The doctor's office had called me back and I was scheduled for another ultrasound that afternoon.

Yesterday we had an embryo, a heartbeat and I was sent home. Today my uterus was empty and the monitor screen for the ultrasound was not even turned for me to see. It was gone. Just like that.

I head home and as I park my car, my phone rings. My doctor calling to talk me through what to expect, and the statistics of it all and that my next pregnancy would be monitored more closely. I want to yell and ask *why wasn't this one monitored as close; doesn't my file have red flags sticking out of it?* My brain tells my heart yelling is unnecessary; it will not bring that baby back.

I was fortunate enough that a D and C was not needed. My embryo had evacuated the premises all on its own. There would be blood work to follow, to check that my body no longer thought it was pregnant. I will get another period, then, following that, we could try again.

Tim shared with me that he was angry. There was no one he could yell at, no one he could fire, nothing he could do. He, again, was helpless.

I realized I was angry too; but I was hurt—and I wanted everyone else to hurt too. Again.

I take the time to cuddle Juliet and contemplate the things I want her to learn from me, compassion tops the list followed by perseverance.

There were no flowers that Valentine's, no romantic dinner, there was wine, however. I drank two very large glasses and did a lot of crying. Everyone else in the world went about their business. Every week I would have blood drawn and later that day get a call about where my level was at and what the next step was. It was clinical and lonely.

We learn later that Tim would not be getting a raise with his company, but a bonus would be coming at the end of the year, which was amazing, but we needed more income now. I have the task in front of me to find work and enough work to be a profit, because now we will also need childcare. Both our families are far away and the siblings that live relatively close to us all have families of their own. The double stressor takes hold.

One night, soon after the miscarriage, with a bit too much wine in me, and too much beer in Tim, I ask him if we should even be trying to have another baby. We are going to let things happen however they do, but, I need a job, and therefore Juliet will need childcare. I did not go through all of that, so that someone else could care for her—but we simply can't afford for me to be a stay at home mom any longer.

It is bizarre how anxious I am about someone else taking care of Juliet; 18 months ago I had no idea how to be a mommy and now I feel as though no one is good enough to take care of this little person. I begin the search online and every site wants money before I commit or they want money before I can contact any viable candidates. Money. The reason we need a babysitter is because we need more money, I don't have any to give away! The other issue is that I only make a few dollars more an hour than the cheapest babysitter. So, whatever income I do make, goes directly to childcare. A cyclical, swirling, drowning situation, why even bother?

Really?

Time passes and Tim goes away for a week on a business trip to Vegas. I get a bad cold, and then give it to Juliet. The solo parenting hardship is compounded when either one of you is sick. In an effort to get into a routine, I decide to utilize my morning time. Juliet has been sleeping through the night for a while, and if I am very quiet I can get up, dressed and head out for a run and sometimes even shower before she wakes up! The days that this works out are great, the days I need my sleep more—I let it go and decide it is a rest day.

Tim's trip has ended and my period is due, and does not show up. I send Tim out for pregnancy tests. The next morning before I take the dog out for our run I pee on the test and very quickly I see the *pregnant* sign. I leave the test on the tank of the toilet for Tim to see when he wakes up.

I decide to walk that morning, instead of run. I can't say that I am in disbelief, but I can say for certain I am not as over the moon ecstatic as I should be. We just had a miscarriage. I think I am trying to protect my heart in case the worst happens again. I keep reassuring myself, just because I don't feel pregnant, doesn't mean I am not. I don't know when I am going to feel blessed and awed. It is not fair to me, in either case. It is not fair to downplay this absolute miracle. It is not fair to expect the bad. What is true, just, and right is that I got a positive pregnancy test. Take the next step.

I call my OB and they send me to get blood drawn. Once again they are measuring my hCG levels. The first one was 977—I know that that is good, and that the goal is for that to double every one to two days. Their protocol is that when I reach around 6,000, I will get an ultrasound. The following blood work is 4,920, I am instructed to go once more and once they get that result, we should be able to go get an ultrasound.

I receive the 4,920 result on my 34th birthday. The night before my birthday I had an episode of self pity. I had not planned any special activities or anything fun to do for myself. My big plan was to do some gardening, make a lovely dinner and a cheesecake and play with Juliet. In reality, that's what I wanted to do, have a normal, regular mommy day. Happiness is a choice, choose to be happy.

My last blood draw of this round results in a 12,119 hCG level. I am instructed to schedule an ultrasound. I am feeling very fatigued lately, and my hips and joints are feeling really tight, even my stomach muscles; like I did too many sit ups or spent the night engaged in a laugh fest. I chalk it up to hormones and all the other stuff you can read about when you are expecting. I still don't feel elated, only anxiety, worry and doubt.

I am able to schedule my ultrasound for the next day at a different location. Tim will go into work late and watch Juliet. They tell me over the phone they have a no children policy. Once there I ask the specifics and I am told that Tim and Juliet can come in the exam room with me, however if she gets fussy or screams, Tim will have to take her out of the room and possibly miss the viewing. So, the policies are crystal clear.

I am called into the romantically lit room. The fluorescents are off, and a stand up lamp in the corner is on, it has soft colored shades making the room feel cozy. She first does an on the belly ultrasound, and right away we see the little sac and a flashing heart beat! She looks some more and seems to be taking data. Then she tells me she will do a transvaginal, to get better pictures and more data. I am asked to put on an enormous hospital gown and remove my underwear and jeans. When I return to the room there is another pillow on the table for my butt. The policy of this radiology group is that the patient puts the wand inside, and then the technician moves it around proceeding with the ultrasound. We chat. It is a relaxed ultrasound, the heart is unmistakable, 136 beats per minute and to me, everything looks good—I am an expert and all. The technician's demeanor is very light and positive, so I figure there is no reason to worry. The baby measures 6 weeks and 6 days, and I am 6 weeks and 4 days—so to me we are right on target. For the miscarriage ultrasound the baby measured 6 weeks and 2 days, but I was in my 7th week at the time. Also, its heart rate was 111, so with that data, I have high hopes for this little one.

I tell my mom the heart rate and her response is,

"Oh, a little boy!"

We'll see if she is right…

I come to the 9 week mark, and finally I get to have a doctor's appointment! I am scheduled at 1:15pm Monday, May 20th, 2013. I have an endocrinology appointment the very next day. I pack up Juliet and myself and head to my OB's office. It is still Dr. Pot Heroin, in case you were worried I would dump her—never, I love her.

I am greeted warmly, and once in the room they have a pregnancy welcome pack for me. A cute pregnancy journal, magazines, and brochures for all the genetic testing, information on cord blood and other overwhelming things.

My doctor comes in, we do a brief once over of results and a quick pelvic exam. Juliet desperately needs a nap and therefore sits on my torso for the exam. Everything checks out and I am to get dressed and meet the doctor in her office for the typical pregnancy chat.

She goes over her well rehearsed routine, all the ins and outs of diet, how many calories I actually need, healthy weight gain numbers and everything else I remember from our first session with her. I confirm that for this pregnancy, like with Juliet's I would not be doing any of the fetal testing for Down Syndrome or anything else. My theory is that I am not going to terminate, so why have months of anxiety about a test result that could be wrong. She tells me she is going to do a quick scan before she sends me home. I hear her in the hall trying to cut in line for the ultrasound room.

We get access to the room, and she performs an ultrasound with Juliet sitting on my chest, screaming. We see a beautiful baby in a black oval; it is clear it has grown since I last saw its image. She very calmly starts trying to get different views, and then says that she cannot see the heartbeat. I too, see emptiness where I have in the past seen a white flicker of magic.

She places blame on the machine and quickly she and her assistant start to call the radiology department across the hospital's campus. They make me an appointment for 3pm, and give me paperwork, water and directions. No one seems too upset, so I don't start to worry—until I call Tim when I reach the car. He tells me he is on his way and I head over to another building.

In the waiting area I do my best to keep Juliet quiet and happy. We are now running on no nap, and no lunch. I had packed her some snacks and water but she wanted neither. Tim arrived and quickly took that burden from me and took her for a walk in the hall and found a vending machine with animal crackers. They return quite happy. Turns out the vending machine itself was a hit.

I am called back and assume the natural state of no clothing from the waist down and a gown, robe style. Quickly, the ultrasound tech also does not detect a heartbeat. She tells me she *is sorry* and she *will make the scan quick*. There is no fetal heartbeat. A beautiful baby inside of my womb, just sitting there. We see it, but there is no life. Only stillness. It is as if it is frozen in space. No gush of blood, no cramping, no sensation of a loss of life at all. I had even felt nauseous that morning. She does finish the images quickly, sadness wells up in my eyes and I desperately wished Tim was in the room.

Once finished she directs me to the restroom and tells me to empty my bladder, get dressed and return to the patient room, she will take the images to the radiologist, call my doctor and we will go from there. Once again, she tells me she is sorry.

I am carrying death inside me. I feel still. Everything around me is business as usual, and I am still and I am alone. The facility is noisy with people and humming with machines and I feel dark, and sad. I feel like I am in the wrong place; I should be in a sunless, boarded up room with silence and other sad people.

I use the restroom to empty my bladder and cry. I know I sobbed loudly, because I caught myself and stopped. I get dressed and head back into the room and I am given a box of tissues. The technician tells me my doctor wants to see me.

I go into the waiting room, with tears and simply shake my head *no* to Tim. I cannot speak. He and Juliet hug me. (She doesn't know what has happened, only that mommy needed a hug.) I finally choke out that we need to go back to my OB. We quickly leave the waiting room, full of people having a normal day. He drives us back over to the other building and we all together go back to her office.

This time we are greeted with an understanding, a sense of sympathy. It was heavy, like everyone knew and metaphorically wrapped their arms around us. It is presented to us that a D and C is appropriate for our situation, also with this procedure the fetal tissue can be tested and we may be able to get an answer for why this happened again. I agree and I am put on the schedule for the next morning. She asks if we had any travel plans for the upcoming Memorial holiday; I am in a wedding in New Jersey. She tells me, I should take some time to think about if I should go; mentally I could be a wreck, physically I will feel like I have a heavy period. We leave the office with our orders, I tell Tim I cannot drive, so we leave my car in the building's garage and use Tim's car to take us all home. I am silent in the passenger seat. Juliet chatters away and Tim responds to her. While at home Tim tells me that my best friend would understand if we cannot go, I tell him I cannot make any decision right now.

Tim orders us pizza, we found a chain that does a very decent gluten free crust. Juliet has her cranky pants on, but I do not hold that against her—she had a rough day too. I call my parents.

"Hello?" My dad answers.

"Hey, it's Mary. There was no fetal heartbeat today…"

"Oh, Mair, I am sorry." He says with a breath of grief. "I'll get mom on the phone."

I recount the day for the two of them. And once again, my parents understand, are loving and ridiculously great in the time of crisis. I guess a nurse and retired cop would have some training in that area.

My dad quickly offers to come down to watch Juliet in the morning while Tim and I are at the hospital. I tell him what a huge help that would be, but I know what a pain in the ass that is for him.

"That's what daddies do."

D and C.

No one but Juliet sleeps that night. The dog is excited a new
person is downstairs on the couch, I cry almost through the night,
Tim comforts me and wakes up almost every half hour worried
that we will oversleep somehow. We need to be at the hospital at
6am, our alarms are set for 4:30am.

I take a shower and cry. While in bed I tell Tim,

"It's not fair."

"No, it's not." He said, simply.

We get to the hospital on time, tired and nervous. Everyone treats
me with kindness. The whole process starts quickly. I am given
two gowns and I smile to myself; there are two in their bags, and
wouldn't you know it, one of them is missing a tie… I make it all
happen and the nurse comes in for the questions and IV prep, and
makes notice that I have not removed my jewelry. I had taken off
my wedding ring, but totally forgot the five piercing in my
ears…I take them out while she asks me routine questions. It is
in my chart, and I noticed right away too, that I am currently
waiting in the same exact room I had prior to my IVF egg
retrieval.

Tim is allowed to wait with me in the pre-op room. We are told
that as soon as the doctor arrives, we will begin. We overhear the
nurses say my doctor is stuck in traffic. I was not allowed to eat
or drink anything past midnight, so I am nervous, hungry and
thirstier than I can ever remember experiencing. The team that
will be with me introduces themselves and we continue to wait.

My doctor arrives and I am escorted to a restroom to empty my
bladder. As we make our way to the OR it gets colder and colder.
We pass what looks like a fridge and my nurse pulls two blankets
out of it. They feel fresh from the dryer. We enter and I see all
the familiar faces. My gown robe is taken, I am instructed to lie
down with my arms out, crucifixion style. My doctor takes my

hand and tells me that they will be able to send the fetal tissue for testing, and in two weeks I will meet with her and we can make a plan. If there were any chromosomal defects, then we will know that there was nothing we could do, and if it was not, then maybe I will need some hormone help, or something else.

My anesthetist begins, the doctor lovingly says,

"He is giving you a cocktail…a mimosa…or whatever morning cocktail you prefer."

"You know, tequila is gluten free." I say

The room laughs and I hear them trying to think up other gluten free alcoholic beverages, and I am quickly sedated, that is the last thing I remember.

A *D and C* is a procedure where the cervix is dilated and the fetal tissue and uterine lining is sucked out. My mom calls it a *Dusting and Cleaning*. There was a list of possible things that could go wrong, and there was paperwork to sign and I was asked if I wanted to submit a living will. There is nothing quite like that question at 6am.

I wake up in the recovery area and feel drowsy and cramped. I am given ginger ale, she apologizes for not having gluten free crackers. Tim is brought back and we begin the process to be released. My pain level is assessed, I am given acetaminophen, I am asked to empty my bladder and once I return the IV is taken out and I am able to get dressed to go home. Everything went well, as planned. I am still drowsy so the full impact of what happened did not hit. We had two miscarriages only three months apart. We now can get pregnant, but not stay pregnant.

We arrive home and a very happy Juliet runs to greet me with her arms spread wide, her smile audible, and her kisses so soft and sweet. My dad tells us how the morning went, and I am proud of my little girl. He gathers his bag and he leaves for NJ as quickly as he had arrived. He didn't sleep well either.

After a meal and a nap I hear from Dr. Pope, my endocrinologist. He had received my news and he offers condolences and shares with me that the fetal tissue testing will be helpful, and that there may be additional testing to see if I am harboring any disorders that may have caused the back to back miscarriages. He also had my most recent blood work and tells me to stay on the same dosage of thyroid medications, and he wants to see me in about six weeks after all the dust settles.

He also tells me, "Hang in there."

Finish smiling.

Am I really going to end this saga with the re-telling of two miscarriages? Did I really have to go through the first trimester crap two more times and still not have a child? Shouldn't there be a happy finale, maybe I should re-write and end with the birth of Juliet. Shouldn't I leave the readers with hope and inspiration—not this, this is all wrong. This is not a normal fertility story! Exactly. So then, this is not a normal fertility story.

I think I may have cried all the tears my body can produce. Describing this feeling as, *sad*, is wrong. Sad is such a small word for an emotion that wrings a body. I promised myself I wouldn't ask *why me*, I wouldn't blame God and I wouldn't forget the happiness I do have. The loss of a pregnancy hurts; physically, emotionally, mentally and spiritually. I don't know the correct way to cope. I know it is not in the half a bottle of wine I drank, and I know it is not in the silent thoughts of *why, how did this happen*?

To cope with this, I need to recognize that I can get pregnant now, I just need help staying pregnant. I have doctors who care, and also want to know why, and how they can help. I do not know what the next chapter is, and that, my friends, is life. I now have had the opportunity to get pregnant with sex, to get pregnant with science, to go into labor and use science to deliver her, to lose a baby in a toilet and to lose a baby surgically evacuated. All these experiences will make me the prime listener for my friends, family and strangers who need a friend.

May 27, 2013

It is a week since the ultrasound showing no fetal heartbeat.

I made a decision earlier in the week that I would allow myself to grieve, but then I would purposely think positively and give myself a fresh start.

My grieving involved a lot of wine. Three large bottles of wine in a matter of five days. I cried a lot, every single day. When I did go out into the world for a short list of groceries, I despised all who were out going about their normal day. They looked so happy, content. I wanted that again.

How to be content after two miscarriages and an IVF baby—do you focus on the baby, what you do have, and not what you want? I am choosing to take it day by day, in fact, moment by moment. A long time ago I wrote out what a perfect day for me would look like. Then I went line by line figuring out how to make it happen. I think I need to employ that tactic again.

In the effort to assess my acceptance and the act of surrender, I commit to thinking *acceptance* and *to surrender* do not mean *to give up*. I don't want to be the woman you need to handle with care. I don't want my newly pregnant friends to hesitate to share their news with me. How did I get here? I want more than anything for people to be careful with what they say and how they say it, but yet, I want to be exceedingly happy for others joy.

The marathon after having Juliet I made it a point to smile, say *thank you* to every officer and volunteer and to be present and happy during the race; to enjoy the race. As the race clocks showed throughout the course that I would not be achieving the pace goal I intended, I decided to keep going, to not give up because I wasn't going to meet my expectations. I kept running, because I wanted to finish, and I wanted to finish smiling. So, that is my metaphor. Yes, I am in pain, but I want to finish smiling.

I go to my follow up appointment two weeks after the D and C. My mental outlook is: *well, I will learn more about what happened and why, and that will help us.* So, needless to say that when I am told that my results are missing, I only sighed. (I smirked inside.) The office is going to continue to make inquiries of the hospital to find them, and in the meantime I am going to be sent home with a lab slip for more blood work. My doctor also asks that I get my fertility doctors involved; check in with them and see if there are any other blood tests that my doctor should order—if there is anything else she is not seeing. I get a bit nervous at this idea. My case nurse left the clinic several months ago for another job and my fertility doctor was recently moved to another office that just opened up in the state. I was unsure as to how exactly I was going to get in touch with anyone. I also feared that this meant we were going to be encouraged to go back to the clinic to conceive. Truthfully, we cannot afford it at all. Also, we had a baby, I don't think I could apply for loans or grants for another one.

I feel guilty. I know Tim and I want another baby, but I feel like I am being greedy. There are days when I feel lousy and I let Juliet watch TV all day. There are days where I just wish the dog would shut up and feed herself. There are days I simply want to stay in my pajamas, drink wine and eat junk. I feel tired. Not the tired I felt when she was just born and I was feeding her every three hours, this tired comes after a full night sleep. I don't stand up straight, I feel heavy, I feel ugly, I feel in a rut and yet the joy I have when I am with Juliet is wonderful. I love her hugs, kisses and the way she responds when learning something new—but even in those bright, shiny moments I feel so far from myself; what is wrong with me?

I receive a voicemail that the results were found and there was a chromosomal problem with our second loss. There was only one X chromosome and this is called Turner syndrome. Apparently a large number of these pregnancies result in miscarriage. I am supposed to find peace in this answer. *Oh, Turner syndrome, why yes, yes, of course that is why I had a second miscarriage.* Once again I find myself doing research on a medical issue that pertains to me. I then wonder if I have Turner syndrome. It must be easy to be a hypochondriac in the age of the internet; you search for something long enough you will find something to support your claim.

I don't actually find peace in this. More like an, *oh well, okay, thanks* type of sigh. Like, when you go to the mall searching for a particular store only to be told by customer information that it closed two years ago. Those kinds of feeling when you feel dumb, lost, and contemplate between going home or seeing what is still there.

I go in for my blood work and they need eight tubes of blood. Eight? That is insane, eight tubes of blood for two tests? What the hell do they think I have? Maybe there is a reason I feel the way I do. Maybe there is a reason for back to back miscarriages.

I am supposed to be pregnant right now. Everything is on hold. We cannot try again until we have more information, hell we even have to use condoms for the first time in years because now we know I can get pregnant, I just can't stay pregnant; at times I wonder if this was the case all along. Though I committed to being positive, the doubt, the distractions, the sulk just creeps in. Again I am in need of reminders as to what helps me not only bring in joy, but helps me stay in joy and peace throughout the day. Mainly, it is all the healthy stuff that keeps me sane and feeling good, but it is the nasty stuff that brings me immediate relief. Sometimes, you just can't go for a run, but having a glass or three of wine is damn simple. Problem is that I feel even more awful later with the wine option. I know I need an alternate remedy.

I begin again. On a Monday I decide to be happy about the day, hell, I am alive, right? I commit to drinking a lot of water (the administrative me even pours out 70 ounces into a pitcher for the fridge so I can keep track). I plan and do a run on the treadmill while Juliet naps. I do the normal household stuff, I also get her to color a Father's Day card for daddy. I find that my focus is…everywhere but where I am. I don't think I am mourning the miscarriages any longer, I am mourning the plan. What was supposed to be; our due date, the rearrangement of the rooms and house, the idea of prepping Juliet, the financial plan, everything that would come next.

There are philosophies that teach on impermanence. The idea that nothing is permanent; we and material things are here for a short while, then gone. With that then, begs the idea of what happened is now over, move on. Is that a healthy approach, or apathy? What is the balance? To enjoy everything in the present,

then when it is gone you happily let it go? Who is even capable
of that? That is why we have 12 step programs, rehab,
bereavement groups, support groups and prayer requests. Or does
all of that simply feed the beast, and not help us move forward?
The weird part is, I came up with all of that without alcohol…

The blood work test results from my eight vials came back
normal. So, now what? I leave a message with my doctor asking
what she suggests I do now. In the meantime once again, I drink
too much wine, and then try to start again with the positive
thoughts. I have a 10 mile race this weekend, and by race I mean
I have paid a registration fee so I can go run 10 miles in
Baltimore with a lot of people I don't know. With the
miscarriages I know I am not in the shape I want to be, I trust I
can cross the finish line but I am not confident I will be able to
run the whole length and know I will walk a portion. There is no
one to blame but myself, and really I am not blaming myself more
like taking responsibility. We are all given the same amount of
time. My circumstances may be different from someone else's'
and that is why I don't *race* necessarily, but finish smiling.

I run the race, and finish smiling and happy. Almost with the
attitude that, well, that is done, what is next? I have (once again)
committed to making some changes. I am not happy, and in order
to move forward I need to make some adjustments.

Since the miscarriages I have felt an overwhelming sadness that is
easy to cover up. I have taken to drinking wine, eating whatever
and whenever I want and wishing myself happy. Talking a good
game, but every breath is a sigh. *Money, debt, I want another
baby* seem to be on repeat. Why not enjoy Juliet, get a job and
get out of debt? If I were an audience member watching this play
that would be the answer I scream from the balcony. Instead I am
hesitating with, *well, it would be so much easier to get pregnant,
have the baby then try to find a job.* What? Really? Are you
dumb? You'll want to stay home with them as long as possible
making it harder on the family financially and putting yourself in
an even harder position to compete in the employment race. Find
a job, start small, maybe part time to not incur day care costs, let

the chips fall where they may and if we stay the course I may be able to carry to term and have baby number 2, then move into full time work. Take care of myself, my family and work—can I do it all? As a stay at home mom I have way more of the house responsibilities, we would need to re-work a lot of that. It will be hard. Life is hard, the task is how will you make sure you enjoy your hard life?

Ah, PMS, we meet again. The first period after the miscarriage. It is surprisingly light, probably because after the D and C it felt like the faucet of blood was perpetually on. My mood is down, down, down in the dumps I feel easily offended and want to be alone. I feel fat and ugly. Yup, I ran a ten mile race two days ago and today I feel fat and ugly. Today I got more done before 10am than most people do and still feel like I accomplished nothing. Hormones are horrible beasts.

So much for it being light! I have been leaking through underwear, jeans, and changing tampons like nobody's business. Ridiculous! Talk about a delayed reaction!

A dear friend is going through IVF. Tonight she triggers. I have been praying for her every day, even before she had her first consultation appointment. I told her I would pray until she was holding that baby of hers. I believe it so strongly that she will be a mommy. I can even see her holding her baby with the typical white, red and blue hospital receiving blanket. I actually also see her husband holding a second baby too—don't know if I should tell her that.

I believe so strongly that she will have a baby, just like I believe so strongly that Juliet will be a big sister one day. It is that vision that keeps me going, the picture of me in the hospital with Juliet and a newborn baby on my lap—smiling and sharing joy.

It is July 2013. My sulking, *woe is me* record plays loudly; I am supposed to be pregnant right now. I tell Dr. Pope about how I have been feeling really tired, have gained weight and feel downright awful. My lab results show everything is normal and he thinks it is time to consult my general practitioner and maybe consider depression as the culprit. He tells me it is going to take some time to heal—that this is big.

I don't want anti-depressants and I don't want to talk to anyone. Talking about it doesn't help, it just scratches the scab, allowing it to bleed. Drinking helps temporarily, but then I pay the price in how I feel and the lack of presence in my awesome life. I think to myself, that here I am once again, alone. I feel like I am silently wading through sludge, going through the business of life in slow motion. How many of us are there? Quietly pushing through life instead of really enjoying it? If I were to play the role of best friend to myself, what advice would I have?

Tricky would understand. She would tell me that it is okay to grieve, that God has never let me down. She would also tell me that this sounds a lot like postpartum depression, and there are drugs that can lift this veil of sadness, and that I deserve to feel that veil lifted.

And, that may not stir me up as much as she wants. Maybe she'll tell me I need more time. Maybe I need a therapist, or medication. Maybe I need a good run. But, I need to seek what it is that I need. I need to seek it as much as I sought help in trying to get Juliet. I need to be relentless. I need to wrangle in my filthy hard working hope ethic and use it to get me better.

Tim comes home late from work and tells me of the HR meeting he had; our health insurance is changing again. We have had the company before, so I am pretty sure all of our current doctors participate—but it is another step for us. I wonder to myself if it is better that we are not pregnant yet… Until he brings home the information packet I have to believe that it will all work out for us.

An early morning text message from my friend undergoing IVF. She had her test today—she is pregnant!

July 17, 2013

I have a new nephew today!

My friend had her first ultrasound and a perfect little yolk sack was seen!

My doctor also got back to me; we have a protocol suggestion. I can track my ovulation, and start progesterone suppositories 3 days after ovulation, (stop if I get a period) and baby aspirin once I am pregnant. I have to call her to confirm that is what we want to do, and we will get started.

I am waiting to talk to Tim tonight before I call her.

Our insurance changes next month, so in theory we could start then. But, I have a marathon in October…but we could also have another miscarriage…but we want another baby…but I only have a part time job and we have debt…

But…I am thinking too much…

What are my motives to getting pregnant? I want Juliet to have a sibling. I want to be a mommy again with a newborn knowing what I know now.

Even so, it feels like daily I think about my faults, failures and question how I am raising Juliet. Hmm, all the things she can't do I blame myself, all the things she can do I give her all the credit. It is a lose lose situation, I am setting my insecurities up; I am not allowing myself the joy of watching her grow.

A prescription of progesterone is at the pharmacy waiting for me.

I told Tim that my doctor called and he was pretty much on board with the whole plan before I even told him what it was. So it seems clear we both want another baby.

I believe it will happen for us, I just don't know when.

In the meantime I land a part time job working once again within the performing arts vein. I can do hours from home, and then be on site on the weekends or the evenings. So, we do not have to struggle with the daycare option yet—I feel blessed and nervous all at the same time. The part time is hourly on a 1099 for the next two months, hopefully after that my boss and the board of directors will see how awesome I am and make me salaried. One day at a time. I feel this job, which really fell into my lap, was a great thing. It gives us more income, relieving some stress of bills, gives me a creative outlet and more daddy daughter time for Tim and Juliet. Also, if we do get pregnant, I will have already been working part time and can we can take life from there.

The week I start I already notice the house work not getting done…but I have also noticed I am consciously more present with Juliet, now to work on my presence in all things. Learning to balance being a stay at home mom and a working mom at the same time is the most bizarre brain melting lifestyle one can engage. The jury is still out if I recommend it or not.

The progesterone has arrived. It is a mixed compound that could not be filled from a standard pharmacy. They are stored in the fridge. They were shipped on dry ice, probably because it is August and they are meant to melt into my insides… Anyway, there were no real instructions on how to preserve them, but if they *get soft, put them in the fridge for a short time*. Okay. That seems very general and random.

The other interesting fact is, these suppositories, I am to shove up my vagina, arrive sans applicators. What the hell am I supposed to do? OB Tampon these suckers up there? Do they even make those tampons anymore? My mom suggested I use rubber gloves. I am more concerned about holding a tiny object and willfully shoving it up my hoo-ha.

My friend's IVF pregnancy resulted in miscarriage. My heart broke instantly. I wept and thought—this is not supposed to happen. She felt the same way. We cried on the phone together, angry at God, saddened by the loss of something so special. Helpless. There is nothing appropriate to say to anyone after a miscarriage. I did a quick search trying to find what the Bible has to say on miscarriage, and well, there are no parables about saint so and so who found herself with multiple miscarriages. It is not fair. I have not known life to be fair. So what do we do? Just expect that this may happen again? How do you hope, when you are prepared for sorrow? What are we praying for exactly? Do I need to get specific and state that I want her and I to get pregnant, carry to term, deliver a healthy baby that lives until old age, succumbs to no tragedy and brings light, joy and peace unto the world? Did I leave any loop holes? Is there a way She can manipulate my prayers so I once again find myself in sorrow? I prayed *thy will be done*, and I regret it. It is not fair. Thy will *not* be done, she is supposed to be pregnant right now.

Another friend has shared she just miscarried. She is in the *we weren't even trying* camp; instantly though, I understood her sorrow and loss. I was not jealous of her conception, and definitely not jealous of her loss. We simply shared our brief story of how the end happened and then moved on to the social atmosphere we were currently in, discussing the onion dip and the humidity as people started to enter the room. Heaven forbid we discuss real human issues that make others uncomfortable at a social gathering. We hide in corners and whisper our tragedies over charcuterie boards and wine.

We need to talk. We need to talk about miscarriages. How come it isn't in the bible? How come it isn't discussed in health class? Why don't we share? Why is it the few, select women who must endure it must also lead the charge of comforter in chief when others do finally share? *...Tricky totally runs a miscarriage support group...*

Talk about your loss. Grieve. Create a mantra for yourself. Accept that a baby will come into your world somehow, some way and surrender to the idea that you will not get what you want when you want it, like all those around you. Allow yourself to cry. Eat sushi, nitrates and lunch meat, drink wine, Long Island iced teas and participate in high impact sports prior to following your strict fertility protocol, whichever yours is. Embrace the experience and learn something from it. Then, once you accept your membership into the infertility, or any other shitty female club, be an advocate, go forth and support another sister.

Hang in there, and cross the finish line smiling.

FINALE

It's not ready yet, it's not in the car.

It is a year after the second miscarriage. I work full time now. I have more infertile friends and I speak openly about IVF whenever possible. We yearn for a *littler one*. Tim and I begin to try again using the ovulation kits and I start progesterone suppositories 3 days after ovulation.

Here is where I get awful. Ugly awful.

My friend finds out at 34 weeks pregnant she has an extremely aggressive form of breast cancer. She has many tests run and it is determined she is to have an emergency c-section at 36 weeks to get the baby out, she will start chemotherapy a mere 10 days later.

I cry and pray for her, offer whatever I can—and it is all truly heartfelt. But here is where I am awful. Her suffering came with a public outpour of support. Her pain is going to be visible with chemo and all the nastiness that comes along with it. A truck load of people will sign up to rush to her aid with overwhelmingly beautiful support. They will think of extra-ordinary and practical ways to help her in this tragic and un-imaginable situation. And she deserves it. She deserves more.

I lost my babies in silence. Alone, barely anyone knew. No physical signs that something was lost. A quiet, internalized pain that I was still feeling a year later. Pregnancy loss is silent, lonely and only shared in hushed embarrassed whispers.

I don't know what to do with those feelings. I feel shitty for feeling them. I wanted comfort. I wanted a train of people telling *me*, it would be okay. I carry on and shove my absurd jealousy and do all that I can for my friend. Later, I will have the unfortunate opportunity to commiserate with yet another friend who suffers a pregnancy loss. I also learn that the train of support my friend with cancer, fades away at the time she needs it most. There is that initial spark of support, but we all selfishly forget to fan the flame for those who need us. We are all terribly ugly at times. We are all selfish, we exhibit it differently.

One night during our normal bedtime routine, I rock Juliet in our rocking chair and we talk about our day. She then proceeds to tell me about how *she did not get to hold her baby yet.*

"It wasn't ready yet". She explained.

Little two and a half year old Juliet then tells me about her two babies that looked just like her though weren't ready yet and she did not get to hold them. But, *they okay, mommy.* She then put her little arm around my shoulder, her head pressed against mine; *I sorry, mommy.* I cried the whole time, every syllable she said, we had never told her about the miscarriages, we thought she was too young.

She then finished her profound stories about the lost babies with:

"I will wait for the next baby, but it's not ready yet, it isn't in the car."

My comfort did not come from a truck load of people lining up to clean my house and hand me casseroles, it came in the way of broken toddler English and her soft hugs and chapped lipped kisses. I told God I needed comfort, and I got it. I got the *I am sorry you didn't get to hold your babies* that I wanted.

Less than a week later I take a pregnancy test. Twice. It is positive. But, no, it is not in the car yet.

I faithfully take my progesterone suppositories and am monitored more closely than before by both my OB and endocrinology. I progress and meet my milestones as a pregnant lady. I throw up all the time. I feel terrible, all the time. I expect a miscarriage all the time. Being a pregnant working mom with a toddler at home is awful, and I think as a nation we need to re-think maternity leave to also include trying to conceive and the duration of pregnancy. We learn we are having a girl and she meets her milestones too. Throughout the pregnancy I worry each day that I will have another miscarriage, and every cramp, even kick feels like it is dangerous. Since I work full time I feel guilty about every moment that I want for myself. I feel so terrible all the time I Google baby girl names that mean *ass kicker*. I find one that immediately is perfect, I text it to Tim (because getting up to walk down stairs to tell him was too much for me to endure) he needs to *think on it*, but I am sure. Within days we have picked out a first and middle name for our *ass kicker gift from God*.

At 35 weeks I wake up one morning and throw up, not out of the ordinary because the morning sickness has still not ceased and I live off of ginger tea, ginger ale and rice. I had even been prescribed Zofran while pregnant to ease the all-the-time-sickness. (Zofran was given to cancer patients to help ease the nausea from chemotherapy, the drug worked for me but has since been proven to be unsafe for pregnant women and it is no longer prescribed in this capacity.) I drink water and sports drink throughout the day and think nothing of my vomit. Tim comes home that night and after dinner, I feel a contraction. Twenty minutes later I get another one, then another like clockwork. Because she is breeched (another breech) and I know I am hydrated, I call the afterhours OB line and explain that I am in labor. The on call doctor calls me back and quizzes me: am I hydrated?…Why did I throw up?…How many contractions?...How far along are you actually?...I tell him that I am coming in, and will have a baby. Apparently, being a parent does indeed make you an obnoxious know-it-all.

I tell Tim we need to go to the hospital. We drive the familiar route. We sign in, this time Juliet joins us in triage and in the tiny exam room. My contractions get closer and are perfectly on time.

We are not ready; there is no hospital bag packed, there is no plan of who is going to watch Juliet while I am in the hospital, there is no work hand off protocol, we are simply not ready. Yet, I am calm, like I am floating out in the ocean, past where the waves break, where it is scary deep, but I have no worries, I am a calm roller girl type goddess, simply taking this all in stride. I look at the clock, it is 9PM on January 4, 2015. I think to myself, if I can hold off for a few hours her birthday will be 1-5-15, that is cool.

That is cool—that is cool, was my honest to God thought about being in active labor that no one else thought was happening. I was in active, pre-mature, dangerous labor with a breeched baby and history of cesarean section. I was the only one in the room who knew (besides the baby) that we were going to have a baby soon.

They give me a dose of medicine to stop the contractions as we stay in the triage room. Tim calls one of my sisters and asks if there is any chance Juliet can stay with her for the night. She drives to the hospital to meet up with Tim for a toddler hand off—I kiss Juliet and ask her to be good to her aunt. I tell her I love her. She confidently leaves my sight, pig tails bouncing.

The contractions ignore the first dose, so they administer another—which is the maximum dosage they can give me of this stop labor drug. The nurse caring for me gives me a knowing look—we are going to have a baby soon, but she has a protocol to follow. I trust her. The on call doctor tells her to try a different drug, I am once again administered the maximum allowed for that one too, and once again, my contractions ignore it. The contractions get closer together and I am finally admitted to the hospital and moved into a large room in the maternity ward.

Though I am admitted there is still zero discussion of the baby and how it will exit my body, and how it needs to be soon.

I do not sleep, I have contractions every five minutes for hours, I am well hydrated so I have to get up and pee many times, however the drugs lower blood pressure, so there is a risk of me falling on my way to the toilet—so I have to ring for a nurse to escort me—every time... I actually wish I had a catheter. I am cold. I am tired. I have to pee. I am in labor. I need to give birth but my cervix doesn't know how and the baby is going the wrong way. And yet, I still feel calm, I know that we will be alright, I do not have fear, I am calmly annoyed.

I never see the on call doctor (literally, he never came to my room or spoke to me or physically examined me), but the nurses, I can tell, are pulling for me and we all know, I need a c-section. I am going to have a baby soon.

I hear a rumor that my OB doctor, Dr. Pot Heroin, goes on call at 9am, and I sigh with relief, surely she will not let these nonsensical stalling tactics continue. The minutes and hours tick by as I lay contracting, cold, feeling anxious, needing to pee...again and again a cycle of *can we get on with this already!*

Travel coffee cup in hand, Dr. Pot Heroin walks into my room in loud disbelief, it is only 35 weeks, it cannot be. She looks at the contraction receipt tape, shakes her head, and tells Tim and me to time the contractions the *old fashioned way*. I am to tell him when they start and end, and he is to time them with a stopwatch. She leaves and we follow orders. One of my nurses comes in, with determination; she rearranges the monitor strap across my belly and says,

"You will get credit for your work."

Tim uses his phone clock and we begin. I tell him when they start, and when they finish. I see color drain from his already pale Irish face.

They are three minutes apart, and within ten total minutes she is back, coffee still in hand...

"Ok, we are having a baby today, I have a scheduled C on the books, and then we will do you." She tells the nurses to prep me and a swarm goes to work.

I exhale relief. The nurses exhale relief. Tim exhales relief.

I am shaved, IV'ed and changed, along with the physical prep; a nurse tells me, *you will not be able to hold your baby, she has to go straight to the NICU, she is premature her lungs are not strong enough.* They are sure to emphasize this part to me, I don't fear this, and in fact I am still calm and confident my *ass kicker* will be alright.

Though the swarm is working there is no sense of urgency, after all there is a scheduled c-section ahead of me. So we wait, Tim calls our parents and I contraction-ally relax.

Then, suddenly, the swarm returns with intense speed, they surround me, and start unplugging me and the gurney is rolling towards the OR. They are jovially chatting and I find myself in the operating room, on the table holding my doctor's hand as I am given the spinal. Turns out the scheduled c-section before me, well the poor thing, she ate applesauce that morning and could not be operated on, so I got bumped up! They almost start cutting me without Tim in the room.

Zelda Jane was brought out into the world and rushed to NICU. She would stay in the hospital for only five days, and it would only be one day before I could finally hold her. The NICU staff nicknamed her feisty Zelda, (I told you she was an ass kicker) and we would learn that this sentiment would stay with her. Though premature she was a great weight and I was able to pump and give her breast milk, thanks to the steam punk industrial breast pumps the hospital keeps in house.

I was released from the hospital the day before Zelda. I was given the option to stay in a room in the hospital overnight, but I chose to go home and sleep one more night before we brought her home. Because of the risk of the cold, flu and RSV, Juliet was not able to see her baby sister in the NICU. It was difficult to go home without a baby, but she was in good care at the hospital. I also went home with a prescription for an antidepressant; which for my postpartum depression proved to be life changing.

Before her release, Zelda had to pass her NICU car seat test; we anxiously hoped her tiny lungs and chest could withstand the seated position for thirty minutes. It was then when I realized what tiny Juliet had said to me before we even knew I was pregnant; *it's not ready yet, it's not in the car.* We brought our double rainbow baby home in the car, and as we entered our home Juliet squealed and happily embraced her little sister for the first time and was ready to enter her new role as *big sister.*

Nothing went as planned. It hasn't since.

July 29, 2018

It is over three years since Zelda's birth. My primary doctor calls me on a Sunday evening, she lets me know my most recent blood work shows that my hormones are in the post menopausal level. I am 39. *(Eh, not too many eggs…)*

I don't know why I cry, I asked for these tests, I knew, I knew, I was going through menopause or something in that change of life realm.

At 37 close to 38 years of age it started with periods that lasted anywhere from ten to fourteen days, then a short break, then another long bleed. I was always bleeding.

Soon the anger began; I would get angry at everything. This was a different anger, it wasn't my jealous rage filled anger, I was fucking livid. I lost my shit at everything. Nothing was too large or too small to make me angry. I would yell, get frustrated and even burst into an audible growl-like grunt when something, anything happened. I also stopped crying. I physically couldn't cry; it was as if all my tears where used up and now I was someone who would get angry instead. It is an anger that you need to apologize for—but don't know exactly how because you feel so utterly justified. It feels rational yet full of self loathing. I never broke chairs or smashed items, but I wanted to. *Menopause anger* is the act of wanting to break every dish in the house, but you don't, because you know, you will inevitably be the one to clean it up so instead you let out a guttural yell. It does not help.

Next came the tossing and turning when I was trying to sleep. The restless leg syndrome-symptoms; I had verbatim what the television commercials described. I could be their spokesperson. Every single night I endured this. I didn't have only the urge to move my legs, but *needed* to, and sometimes *needed* to scratch them too. I felt like I understood an addict going through detox.

Soon the hot flashes; which everyone equates with menopause but no one ever describes exactly what it feels like. It felt like I was extremely embarrassed and suddenly sweaty at inopportune times. A rush of embarrassing flushing would rush through my arms, legs, chest and face and nothing could remedy it. At the time, I thought I was crazy, I had no idea what was happening, it felt like a physical panic attack—so that is what I treated it as. I combined it into my anxiety and post partum depression symptoms.

Night sweats actually happened at night, when I could sleep I would wake up startled, as if from a bad dream, and then realize I was soaking wet. I would physically change my pajamas including underwear, and sometimes put a towel on top of my soaked side of the bed and change the sheets in the morning. I would try to fall back asleep. At first I thought I must have a fever. But I never had a high temperature and it happened several times a week.

And then my periods stopped for several months and I accepted the change. But, then, unexpectedly, they appeared, though in a very different manner than their former selves; they were light, spotting and did not even require a feminine supply. Then without any fanfare, they completely stop.

Finally, the pooch appears. Even though I run and do yoga every day a pouch of a belly appears, where I would keep my joey if I were a kangaroo. I think it is bloating, and then resign that maybe this is just what my post baby body looks like.

When I spoke to my primary doctor, I suggested I was going through menopause. I was met with disbelief (*but you are so young*) but understanding; she realized my symptoms were real to me and that I was seeking relief. She ordered a large panel of hormone checking tests. However, whenever I brought up to anyone that I thought I might be experiencing menopause the automatic response was, *no, you are too young for that.* Says fucking who?

So when the tests results came in, they were exactly what my brain expected, but I still wept. I cried not at the loss of my fertility, but at the unfairness. (Finally, I was able to cry though!) My primary care physician and Dr. Pot Heroin decide on a low dose estrogen—*again with the birth control pills*, an anti depressant, along with my thyroid medication, and additional iron would round out a daily pill regimen I keep in a plastic flip top days of the week pill box, like old people have. The estrogen helps but it takes several months to kick in. I start to educate myself on foods for menopausal women and make the appropriate additional diet changes. I found that adding salt helps my restless legs. I also try intermittent fasting and that helps the kangaroo pouch a bit. My rage and emotions are never consistent; sometimes I am sluggish and lethargic, other days I am extremely productive and clear. The night sweats come and go, but the hot flashes have altogether stopped after adding the estrogen. I am encouraged to lose a bit of weight because it will create an optimal environment for the estrogen to continue to help. I find the best fit of an anti-depressant but still need to daily keep my mind healthy. I do this with journaling, meditation, yoga, runs outside and reading. Binge watching shows and eating junk doesn't help, so I do my best to stop doing that even though it is exactly what I want to do.

I am a hot mess mom of two. I own my hot mess-ness. My girls are wickedly smart, funny and beautiful. They are my breathtaking shooting stars worth every tear I shed. They changed me. I now abstain from both alcohol and caffeine and routinely go to bed early. I teach yoga, run every day, and my husband and I own a business in the entertainment industry. I have completed five full marathons and run at least two long distance races a year. However, there are days I am so anxious I wonder if I even do self care wrong. Every day my goal is to fail my girls in the least detrimental way possible, and every day I surprise myself. There are moments I think *this is why conceiving was so hard*, my insecure self thinks I am not cut out to be a parent. Then, the girls will ask to listen to Queen, or read Harry Potter and I think, ok, I am not that terrible at helping little humans develop… They have had to bear the brunt of my menopausal ups and downs and it gives us an opportunity to share our feelings. I can't hide from them, and hiding what we go through is bad for our mental health. Our family hones gratitude daily by simply sharing with each other our favorite part of the day. This one simple habit became the roots of our family.

I have reigned in the Jealousy, realizing that one should never be jealous of someone unless you are one hundred percent ready to go through whatever they did to get it. Now, I know what you are thinking, *but so and so wasn't even trying to get pregnant*… yes, it isn't fair. But, there is some trial in her life that you do not know about, and by accepting the unfairness, and embracing the shit storm you are in is a whole lot easier than filling yourself up with Jealousy, Rage and Hate. You don't have to attend her baby shower, and you don't have to be thrilled for her. You do have to give yourself a break, and allow some room for hope in that head and heart of yours. What grows is what you feed. Feed your hope. That may mean you need some space, or a social media break, or therapy. Hope looks different. Mine was filthy. But feed your hope and don't apologize if it is inconvenient for those around you. Your growth will make people uncomfortable. So, if avoiding a baby shower feeds your hope, then own that. If creating a *trying to conceive* social media account feeds your hope, then own that. If reading every book about fertility feeds your hope, then own that. But check in, daily, to ensure you are feeding and cultivating hope (or whatever positive word you choose) with truth. Take the tests, learn the facts, engage with truth and if it aligns with your hope, then you are on a perfect path. Remember, normal for one is not normal for all.

Your baby is going to come, somehow, some way, and it won't be the picture perfect plan you thought it would be. Exhaust every possibility. Be open to all the advantages and disadvantages in front of you. Share your feelings, experience and fears. We need to talk to each other. We need to normalize this. All of it, infertility to menopause—we need to normalize women. You are not the first woman who has ever seen a negative pregnancy test. You are not the first woman to have miscarried. You are not the first woman to gush an embryo into the toilet. You are not the first woman to hear the diagnosis of *unexplained infertility*. You are not the first woman or couple to experience this ugly mess. You are not the first woman who felt the need to smile and nod when told that *just relax* was a method of conception. You are not the first woman to be dismissed when you have a gut feeling that something is wrong. We live in such isolated minds that we think we are shamefully alone. There is no shame with infertility, zero. Speak up, listen up, ask, learn and do all that the crisis demands, then, allow it change you for the better.

I still have a *Tricky Cervix* aspiration. I have been pierced and tattooed, scarred and strong, earthy, hippy and kind. There are many days when balance and acceptance are out of reach and on those days, I ask for help, and I do not apologize for my existence. When it comes down to it, we all have that strong woman alter ego in there somewhere who can summon all the courage and strength necessary to do whatever is to be done, and we all need to be each other's strength when our *sister* gets too overwhelmed. You are not alone.

I strongly ask that we normalize infertility, miscarriage, pregnancy loss and menopause. Let's break the cycle. I respectfully ask that if this book helped you in any way, that you share it with someone who may benefit from it.

I also humbly ask that you go to Amazon and post a review of this book. An honest one. This was a self published labor of love with the sole purpose to write the book I wished I had access to when I was trying to conceive. Self published authors do not have the benefit of large marketing budgets or corporate backing, so we rely on submitted reviews and internet word searches. Reader reviews are the best way self published authors can gain exposure, help sales and spread their message.

If you need support from me or others you can find *Tricky Cervix* on Instagram and Facebook: @Trickycervix.

I am here, because you are not alone.

Thank you, I am rooting for you to finish smiling, whatever your race is.